Milady's SKIN CARE AND COSMETIC INGREDIENTS DICTIONARY

Natalia Michalun
with
M. Varinia Michalun

Milady Publishing Company
(A Division of Delmar Publishers Inc.)
3 Columbia Circle, Box 12519
Albany, New York 12212-2519

NOTICE TO THE READER

Publisher does not warrant or guarantee any of the products described herein or perform any independent analysis in connection with any of the product information contained herein. Publisher does not assume, and expressly disclaims, any obligation to obtain and include information other than that provided to it by the manufacturer.

The reader is expressly warned to consider and adopt all safety precautions that might be indicated by the activities described herein and to avoid all potential hazards. By following the instructions contained herein, the reader willingly assumes all risks in connection with such instructions.

The publisher makes no representations or warranties of any kind, including but not limited to, the warranties of fitness for particular purpose or merchantability, nor are any such representations implied with respect to the material set forth herein, and the publisher takes no responsibility with respect to such material. The publisher shall not be liable for any special, consequential or exemplary damages resulting, in whole or in part, from the readers' use of, or reliance upon, this material.

Credits:
Publisher: Catherine Frangie
Developmental Editor: Laura V. Miller
Art/Design Supervisor: Susan C. Mathews
Production Manager: John Mickelbank
Freelance Project Editor: Gail Hamrick
Cover Design by: design M design W

© 1994 Milady Publishing Company
(A Division of Delmar Publishers Inc.)

For information address:

Milady Publishing Company
(A Division of Delmar Publishers Inc.)
3 Columbia Circle, Box 12519
Albany, NY 12212-2519

Printed in the United States of America
Printed and distributed simultaneously in Canada

3 4 5 6 7 8 9 10 XXX 00 99 98 97 96 95

Library of Congress Cataloging-in-Publication Data

Michalun, Natalia.
    Milady's skin care and cosmetic ingredients dictionary / Natalia Michalun with M. Varinia Michalun. — 1st ed.
        p.   cm.
    ISBN 1-56253-125-5
    1. Cosmetics—Dictionaries.   I. Michalun, M. Varinia.   II. Title.
III. Title: Cosmetic ingredients dictionary.
TP983.M498   1994
668'.55'03-dc20

                                                            93-33822
                                                            CIP

CONTENTS

CONTENTS

Thank you also to Elaine R. Dock, Kathleen L. Driscoll, Cindy French, and Mark Lees for their expertise and very helpful input while reviewing this manuscript.

Although this book does not specifically address body and hair care cosmetic ingredients, we hope it provides the answers to the many skin care cosmetic ingredient questions that estheticians and cosmetic consumers have.

Delmar Publishers' Online Services

To access Delmar on the World Wide Web, point your browser to:

http://www.delmar.com/delmar.html

To access through Gopher: gopher://gopher.delmar.com

(Delmar Online is part of "thomson.com", an Internet site with information on
more than 30 publishers of the International Thomson Publishing organization.)

For information on our products and services:

email: info@delmar.com

or call 800-347-7707

themselves. This book intends to provide the reader with the tools necessary to achieve this understanding.

Although this book is the result of many months of research by its authors, it really is a compilation of the work and knowledge of many people who, through time, have contributed to the growth and the development of the U.S. esthetics and cosmetic industry. What we present in this book is the result of their efforts and their help.

It is impossible to acknowledge everybody who has made this industry and our book possible. However, there are some individuals and organizations that have been essential to us. My very special appreciation goes to Mrs. Christine Valmy, whom I consider the "Mother" of the esthetics industry in the United States. I was introduced into this industry through her, and her teaching, dedication, and high standards of scientific and technical understanding have guided my career over the years.

We want to thank the Allured Publishing Corporation for publishing their outstanding magazine, *Cosmetics & Toiletries,* that has been the best source of reference we have found for all our research on cosmetic ingredients. Our thanks to the many wonderful cosmetic chemists and technical support people from different companies who so willingly and generously cooperated with us, especially Mr. Peter Cade at Croda, Mr. Stephen Greenberg at Lipo, and Mr. Jim Burroughs at Hormel.

For botanical descriptions, we found the two volumes of *A Modern Herbal* by Mrs. M. Grieve as probably the most complete and comprehensive work available to date. Other sources we have used include Dr. Michael Weiner's *Weiner's Herbal,* Mr. Marcel Lavabre's *Aromatherapy Workbook,* William A.R. Thomson, D.M.'s, *Guia Practica Ilustrada de las Plantas Medicinales,* and *Dermascope* and *Les Nouvelles Estetiques* esthetics magazines.

Finally, our heartfelt thanks to Dr. Roger P. Friedenthal for reviewing Part I and to the cosmetic chemistry professionals, estheticians, esthetics instructors, and laypeople who looked over the material and provided their valuable input.

FOREWORD

I have been teaching advanced skin care concepts and technologies to esthetics professionals for many years. One of the most popular subjects has always been cosmetic chemistry, including cosmetic ingredients and the understanding of product labels. In the course of my teachings, both in the United States and abroad, I have seen the looks of great bewilderment that cross my students' faces when they are presented with unfamiliar chemical names. At the same time, I have also seen the desire to understand these confusing names, government regulations, and cosmetic naming and labeling practices adopted by companies for regulatory and marketing reasons.

This is a time of great new developments in the cosmetic industry. It is also a time of professional and consumer savvy and skepticism about marketing claims made by cosmetic companies. Estheticians, together with their clients and the general cosmetic consumer, are increasingly concerned about the value and performance of the ingredients present in cosmetic products. People want to know (and justifiably so) what to expect of the products they are using. If no one can tell them or give them a satisfactory answer, they are more and more seeking ways to find out for

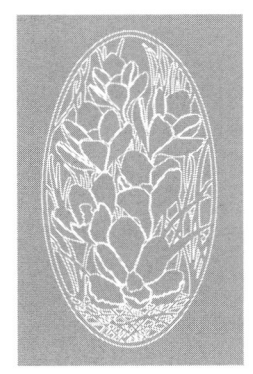

Part I
THE SKIN

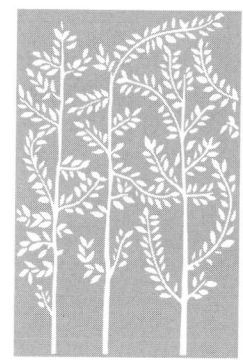

INTRODUCTION

Cosmetic products without the human skin have no purpose. Their value, efficacy, function, virtues, and problems are valid only within the framework of the skin they are supposed to beautify and enhance. To give cosmetics, especially skin care products, any value, it is important to understand how the products work on the skin, what function or functions they perform, what problems they solve, and how the skin may react to them. Without this understanding, the use of skin care cosmetics remains a mystery, for some translated into "hope in a jar" and for others the "miracle solution" to a multitude of skin problems. The first step to solving the mystery of skin care product performance is by asking two basic questions: What are cosmetics? And, what can they be expected to do?

By strictest definition cosmetic products are those that remain on the surface of the skin. More loosely defined, skin care cosmetic products are those that penetrate the top layer of the skin (the corneum layer), and in some cases the epidermal tissue, but do not reach the skin dermis and are not absorbed by the blood capillaries located in this second layer. Products that penetrate the dermal layer and are absorbed by the capillarian system are classified as pharmaceuticals and are subject to Food & Drug

3

INTRODUCTION

Administration (FDA) safety requirements. In practical terms, cosmetic products are those that are formulated for the beautification of the skin, making no claim of performing in a drug related fashion.

Cosmetic products can perform in a variety of ways. They can:

1. remain strictly on the skin's surface

    a) for occlusion (holding together or closing) of the top layers of cells. This favors skin hydration by reducing moisture loss—a very important factor for avoiding dehydration and accelerated skin aging.

    b) for protection against ultraviolet (UV) radiation, thereby also reducing skin aging and skin cancer incidence.

    c) to balance the skin's pH (or acid mantle), which may help control surface bacteria population. This may be an important factor for very oily and acne skins, since excessive bacteria population is one of the main conditions that appears to aggravate acne.

    d) to heal the wounds caused by acne.

    e) to soften the top layers of dead cells and facilitate their removal. This helps give the skin a softer, smoother texture.

2. penetrate the top epidermal layer or corneum layer to

    a) facilitate skin hydration by introducing hydrating ingredients into the intercellular channels.

    b) form a so-called reservoir or "time-release capsule" (as with liposomes) from which moisture or special ingredients may slowly be released into the corneum layer and/or the epidermis.

    c) favor deep exfoliation by softening the cohesive bonds that glue the corneum cells together.

3. penetrate into the pilosebaceous orifice for

    a) regulating oil gland secretion.

NOTE: Throughout the following chapters a large number of the skin's chemical components and other technical terms will be introduced. They have been purposely presented and/or discussed to familiarize the reader with the new terminology used by cosmetic chemists, which is also being incorporated into new product formulations. For definitions of some of these terms, see chapter 4.

development of acne. Lack of sufficient oil secretion is associated with skin dryness.

Sweat glands are abundant over the whole skin with high concentrations in the axillae (armpits), the palms of the hands, the soles of the feet, and the forehead. Each gland begins in the dermal tissue as a coiled end. It continues as a single excretory tube or duct through the epidermis and finally opens on the surface as a very tiny pore.

It is important to note that dirt, impurities, and the asphyxiation, or clogs, seen in the pores occur in the hair follicle. They are the result of a mixture produced by the oil and the keratinized, or corneocyte, cells present in the follicle. Cleansing the skin means eliminating impurities from these pores. **Perspiration is not a cleanser.** It may help clean the minute openings of the sweat pores, but perspiration will not cleanse the pore made by the hair follicle—the pores through which oil is secreted. This is a regular misconception by those who feel that saunas or perspiration through exercise cleans their skin.

The secretion of oil and sweat mixed together on the skin's surface forms the pH balance, or skin's protective mantle. The normal pH of the skin is between 5.6 and 6.6, depending on the skin condition and the place on the body from which the reading is taken. Though not a universally accepted concept, in some circles it is believed that skin acidity helps reduce bacteria populations.

All of these components are found within the basic building block of skin tissue, treated and discussed as three layers.

THE SKIN'S LAYERS

The surface of the skin, the part visible to the naked eye and upon which cosmetic products are applied, is made of a conglomeration of dead cells. Underneath the surface, the skin's multiple functions take place over three very thin and distinct layers made of different skin tissues—the epidermis, the dermis, and the hypodermis. (Fig. 1.1)

The epidermis is very thin. Its thickness varies from 1.6 mm on the soles of the feet to 0.04 mm on the eyelids. The Langerhans skin is not in harmony because of deterioration due to age, sun damage, bacteria infection, hyperkeratinization, or simply loss of natural moisture, cosmetic products are meant to assist in restoring balance and beauty. They must do so, however, by working in conjunction with the skin's very complex structure.

THE SKIN'S COMPONENTS AND STRUCTURE

The skin has a very intricate microanatomical structure. Within one square inch of skin, varying from 1mm to 4mm in thickness, there are some 650 sweat glands; 65 hair follicles; 19 yards of capillaries; 78 yards of nerves; and thousands of sensory cells, nerve endings, and Langerhans cells. The skin also contains melanocyte cells and the tyrosinase enzymes, responsible for producing the melanin that gives the skin its color and pigmentation spots, or freckles. For a solid visual understanding and a bit of challenging fun, draw a one-inch square and in it attempt to make 650 dots representing the sweat pores. Then take a spool of thread, measure 19 yards, and place it within the square. If you're having a hard time with 650 dots and 19 yards of thread, imagine trying to add 1,300 nerve endings and 78 yards of nerves! All of this is found in one square inch of skin, about as thick as a few stacked sheets of paper.

Two types of glands are housed within the skin: oil glands and sweat glands. These glands are important not only because of their intrinsic functions but because they represent a route of entry into the skin for certain chemical compounds.

Oil glands, responsible for oil secretion in the skin, are held within little sacs. The ducts of the oil gland open into the upper portion of the hair follicle. Usually there is only one oil gland per follicle, but in some locations there may be more, which results in greater oil (sebum) secretion in that area. Oil glands are found in almost all parts of the body. The face and back contain the highest number per square inch of skin, while the palms of the hands and soles of the feet contain none.

The sebum lubricates the skin and helps prevent the evaporation of moisture. Excessive oil secretion is associated with the

Cosmetic products become very important to this protective function. Sunscreens protect against UV radiation and therefore against premature skin aging and skin cancer. Creams and lotions with a bactericidal effect reduce and/or control excessive proliferation of bacteria on the skin, a problem particularly associated with oily skin and one of the main causes of acne development. And, by forming an invisible barrier on the skin's surface, daytime moisturizers can help reduce the moisture lost by the skin itself that results in dehydration.

Through the secretion of sweat and sebum, the skin performs an excretory function, eliminating a number of harmful substances resulting from the metabolic activities of the intestine and the liver. The skin also secretes hormones and enzymes. When the skin's own chemistry and chemical composition are not compatible with a particular product's ingredient(s), the result is overall product sensitivity and even allergic reactions.

The large number of nerve endings in the skin makes it sensitive to touch. As a result the skin is a sensory organ and the point of receptivity for cold, heat, and pain.

Finally, the skin plays an immunological role, due primarily to the Langerhans cells that can pick antigens from the skin and carry them to the lymph nodes. Excessive UV radiation either destroys or inhibits the performance of these cells, increasing the risk of skin cancer.

The skin tends to be discussed and treated as an entity unto itself, so this close relationship between the skin and the body is often overlooked or forgotten. Though it protects the body in a variety of ways, the skin and its condition is governed by a number of internal body functions. For example, skin oiliness arising from oil gland overactivity and pigmentation problems due to the tyrosinase enzyme are regulated by hormonal functions. This connection to the rest of the body highlights the importance of proper nutrition, exercise, and rest for the best appearance of the skin. It also highlights the potential problems that ingredients penetrating deep into the dermis may cause if they are systemically absorbed by the capillary system.

When the skin performs in perfect harmony, the result is a beautiful, glowing, healthy skin surface, or complexion. If the

Chapter 1
SKIN PHYSIOLOGY

The skin is a magnificent, complex, multipurpose organ. But it is not completely understood. More has been discovered about the way the skin functions and its components and structure in the last ten years than in the last two hundred. This increase in knowledge allows us to see the direct and indirect relationship between skin care cosmetic product performance and skin physiology.

THE SKIN'S FUNCTIONS

As the body's largest organ, the skin performs a series of key functions resulting from multiple chemical and physical reactions taking place within it. The most common and obvious of these functions is to protect the body against injury, heat, and light radiation; the penetration of chemical agents; and the invasion of microbes and microorganisms. The skin also acts as a temperature regulator, enabling the body to adapt to different ambient temperatures and atmospheric conditions by regulating moisture loss.

The epidermal cells are formed in the germinative layer and move upward toward the corneum layer. In their upward process, epidermal cells undergo a number of chemical modifications, transforming from soft, protoplasmic cells into flat surface "scales" that are constantly being rubbed off.

The epidermis holds a large amount of water. The layer with the highest water content is the germinative layer, holding about 80%. Each subsequent layer has less water as a percentage of its total chemical composition, with the corneum layer containing only 10–15% water. Water is held in the cell's cytoplasmatic gel and in the intercellular channels (spaces between the cells). The younger the body, the more water there is in the skin. The skin's capacity to retain water decreases with age, making the skin more vulnerable to dehydration and wrinkles.

In a young person it takes approximately twenty-eight days for a cell to travel from the germinative to the corneum layer. With age, the speed of this process is greatly reduced. It is estimated that after the age of fifty, it takes about thirty-seven days to complete the same process. Put in terms of skin aging, this indicates that stimulating skin functions, either manually through facial massage or through cosmetic product activity, would improve cellular metabolism. The twenty-eight and thirty-seven-day time span is also important when it comes to skin sensitivity and the misuse of facial scrubs. If it takes twenty-eight days or more for a cell to reach the surface of the skin, then we are naturally exfoliating one layer of dead cells a day. At times, often because of excessive oiliness, we may accumulate a few extra layers. Depending on the harshness of the material, the use of scrubs may remove more layers of surface dead cells than appropriate for the skin. As a result, excessive use of facial scrubs (especially if harsh) may increase skin sensitivity. Furthermore, the misuse of scrubs may exacerbate oil gland activity, increasing oil production—the opposite of what the user generally wishes to achieve.

Epidermal Layers. Understanding the epidermal layers allows us to comprehend the problems of dehydration, sensitivity, aging, and pigmentation, which in turn helps associate product and ingredient effectiveness with skin requirements. The cells of the four epidermal layers from the germinative to the lucidum layer are referred to as keratinocytes and are the predominant cell species found in the epidermis. It is now believed that the primary function of the keratinocytes is manufacturing the uppermost layer—the corneum layer. An improperly functioning keratinocyte formation system cannot generate a cosmetically acceptable corneum layer. Hence, an important factor for beautiful skin appears to be the appropriate metabolism of keratinocytes in order to generate a healthy corneum layer.

The germinative layer, also referred to as the basal layer, is where the cells reproduce by subdivision—one cell dividing into two, identical to one another and to the original parent cell. A healthy and active germinative layer results in a youthful and compact skin surface. After subdivision, one cell remains in the basal layer and the other is pushed upward toward the mucosum layer. In young skin the germinative layer is the thickest layer of the epidermis. Here the cells are large and supple and contain a high percentage of water. With age this layer thins, making it difficult for the skin to retain moisture. The lipids present in this cellular stage are mainly phospholipids.

As the cells move upward, they begin to fill with a granular substance called keratin (hence the term *keratinocyte*), lose water, and flatten. In the subsequent layers, the granulosum and the lucidum layers, the cells are increasingly filled with keratin fibers and contain considerably less moisture. The lipid composition, initially of phospholipids, begins to change in the granulosum layer, showing glycolipids, as well as cholesterol and ceramides.

In their last stage of migration, the cells reach and form the corneum layer (also referred to as the stratum corneum). Traditionally, this layer was viewed merely as a layer of dead cells. Today, it is considered so important and critical to product penetration, skin hydration, and the reduction of skin sensitivity, that it is often studied apart from the other epidermal layers. The corneum layer, or cornification of the keratinocytes, is what we see as our skin. It is made of eighteen to twenty-three layers of flattened, dry cells (corneocytes) firmly cemented together. The actual number of layers depends on the amount of oil in the skin. Oily skin will tend to have more layers than dry skin, making oily skin look thicker and coarser while dry skin looks thin. The corneum layer is almost fluidless, retaining only some 10–15% of its original moisture. Its principal activities are to prevent excessive dehydration of the skin tissues and prevent foreign matter from penetrating the skin. The cells are held together and surrounded by lipids and ceramides, plus glycoproteins, dermasomes, peptide breakdown products, sebaceous products, and active enzymes. This material is usually referred to as cellular cement. The intercellular lipids play a crucial role in the skin's water retention properties by acting as a barrier, trapping water, and preventing excessive water loss.

Ceramides account for up to 40% of the total intercellular matter and also play a vital role in the skin's water balance. They have a great ability to repair the skin's water-retaining capacity, which is often damaged from aging and sun exposure.

The corneum layer includes a natural moisturizing factor (NMF) made of hydrosoluble (able to dissolve in water), hygroscopic (able to retain water) substances that regulate the corneum's selective permeability. The NMF is composed of about 40% free amino acids, some 12% PCA, 12% lactose, 7% urea, and approximately 30% of a large variety of other materials. Exposure to harsh detergents and climatic conditions can result in decreased NMF levels, rendering the skin fragile and dry.

The thickness of the corneum layer, the appropriate arrangement of its cells on the skin's surface, and the strength of the cellular cement greatly determine a product or ingredient's ability to penetrate. When the corneum layer is thin and its cells are arranged in a scaled, uneven pattern, the natural barrier action of the skin is reduced, allowing for faster substance penetration. This is one of the reasons why products give a burning sensation when the skin is very dry and scaly. When the skin is excessively moist, sensitivity also may occur because the "barrier" has been softened, resulting in increased ease of product penetration.

The proper balance of all the epidermal elements is essential for the appropriate functioning of keratinocytes and the corneum layer. Without such a balance the beauty of the skin is impaired.

The Dermis

The second layer of the skin, much thicker than the epidermis, is the dermis. This layer serves two principal functions. One is the nutrition of the epidermis by means of its vast network of capillaries and blood vessels. The second is the formation of a supporting framework composed of collagen and elastin protein fibers. (Fig. 1.2) The dermis is responsible for skin's elasticity.

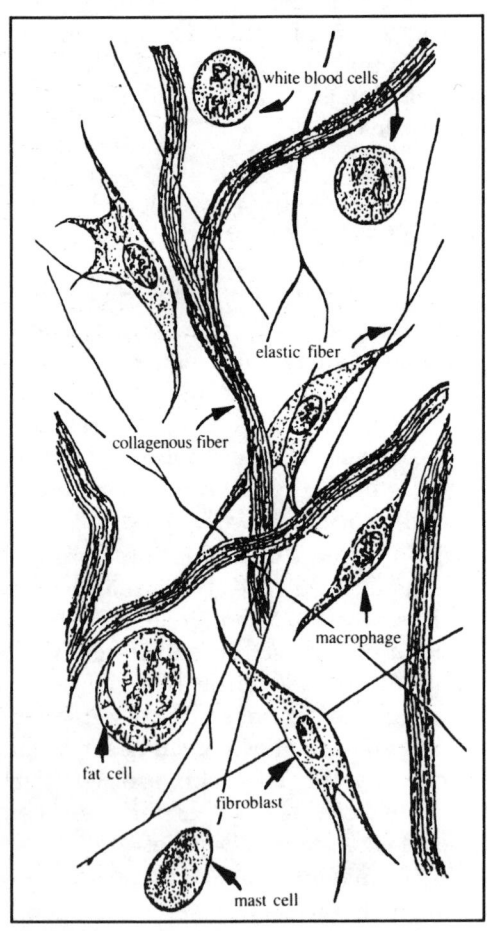

FIG. 1.2 Dermal fibers *(courtesy of Geo. A. Hormel and Co.)*

This elasticity depends greatly on a well-balanced water content in the dermis and other skin layers.

The dermis consists of a thick connective membrane crisscrossed by blood vessels, lymphatic vessels, nerve fibers, and many sensory nerve endings. Collagen and elastin protein fibers, the two main components of the dermis, act as a structural support system for the nerve fibers, hair follicles, blood vessels, oil and sweat glands located in this layer and also provide the skin with strength and elasticity.

Collagen is the dermis' principal component and is basically a chain of amino acids including alanine, arginine, lysine, glycine, proline, and hydroxyproline. Its production begins with the elaboration of procollagen, which later undergoes a series of modifications and is transformed into regular collagen. Procollagen is very hygroscopic and binds many times its weight in water. A decreasing procollagen content during aging may be related to the increased dryness and lack of elasticity associated with mature skin. Similarly, the water-binding capacity of collagen is reduced and the skin loses its elasticity with advancing age.

How elastin is formed in the dermis is not yet fully understood. The first stage is the formation of soluble proelastin that, after a series of reactions, is transformed into fibrous elastin.

Filling the space between collagen and elastin are glycoproteins, forming something akin to a protective mantle. Among these glycoproteins are glycosaminoglycans and fibronectin. Glycosaminoglycans are a fundamental dermal material providing support, lubrication, and the proper environment for the development of dermal cells. They also have a great water-binding capacity and hence are crucial for the healthy turgor (normal distention), water content, and elasticity of the skin. Although they are sometimes referred to as mucopolysaccharides, they are not exactly the same material. Mucopolysaccharides are a component of glycosaminoglycans. Fibronectin appears to be another important dermal component. A glycoprotein of high molecular weight, fibronectin is increasingly considered important for fibroblast growth.

The proper functioning of the dermal layer, as well as its water content, accounts for the skin's smoothness and elasticity.

A properly functioning dermis is key for a youthful appearance and beautiful skin.

The Hypodermis

The hypodermis, the skin's third and last layer, connects the skin with the muscle tissues. The hypodermis may be regarded as the extension of the strong fibrous and elastic bundles forming the dermis. This layer is highly elastic and has fat cells acting as "shock absorbers," thus supporting delicate structures such as blood vessels and nerve endings.

The skin, with its many tiny components and multilayered structure, is staggeringly complex. For the skin to be healthy and beautiful, balance and the proper working of all interrelated elements is essential. As more light is shed on how the skin works, cosmetic chemists have new elements to consider when exploring improvements in the functioning of different skin mechanisms.

The cosmetic chemist's concerns include:

- how biochemical reactions might alter the conversion of keratinocytes into a corneum layer cell
- how to maintain the corneum layer's optimal appearance
- how to preserve or augment its barrier function
- how to improve the dermal layers, presumably the sites responsible for skin wrinkling and sagging

Augmenting the challenge to the cosmetic chemist is that this must be done within the established guidelines defining cosmetics and product penetration.

Chapter 2
PRODUCT
PENETRATION

Cosmetic product penetration, how it happens, why it happens, and whether it happens, has been a subject of much concern, confusion, and debate. This is true not only among product consumers, but in industry circles as well. Until recently it was believed that the corneum layer was impenetrable. The world was once considered to be flat. Beliefs change; discoveries are made. It is now considered common knowledge that products or their ingredients do penetrate to varying degrees. The world is round.

A change in awareness exposes the issue at hand, in this case cosmetic product penetration, to a whole new set of questions. How do products penetrate? Is penetration important for skin care cosmetic product efficacy? Is product penetration crucial for actual cosmetic treatment of specific skin types and conditions?

We can begin answering these questions by clearly understanding the defined parameters of product penetration, including the whys and hows, plus factors that could affect it.

WHAT IS PRODUCT PENETRATION?

By definition, product penetration is the movement of substances or chemicals through the skin. The goal of a cosmetic product is to adhere or bind to the upper layers of the epidermal corneum layer with little or no absorption of the "active" cosmetic ingredient(s) into the skin. Product absorption into the skin falls within the realm of pharmaceuticals.

With the current concern that true efficacy is based on a variety of product attributes, particularly penetration, it must be remembered that the skin's health and beauty can be benefited even with surface activity of the therapeutic ingredients present in skin care products. Such products include cleansing treatments, protective moisturizers, and sunscreens. Products intended to heal acne blemishes, balance surface pH, reduce bacteria population, reduce hyperkeratinization, and reduce moisture loss are all designed and formulated for surface performance. These types of products work best if absorption is minimal. Penetration, therefore, may remove significant quantities of the therapeutic ingredient from the skin's surface, thereby reducing and even eliminating product efficacy.

WHY PRODUCTS PENETRATE

Product penetration may be attributed to one or more of a variety of reasons including the condition of the corneum layer, the molecular size of the compounds involved, the density of hair follicles and the pilosebaceous orifice, the health of the individual, and where the product is applied.

It is clear that the skin's ability to serve as a barrier is largely dependent on an intact corneum layer. Removal or alteration of this layer from either scraping, scaling (due to dryness), application of products like Retin-A™ or alpha hydroxyacids, or skin diseases such as eczema and psoriasis may increase penetration.

Movement through the corneum layer depends on the molecular size of each ingredient and their tendency to metabolically interact. If movement through the corneum layer is slow, a significant concentration of the product will develop. This results in a reservoir-like situation where the corneum layer holds that which has penetrated and supplies the underlying tissues with a particular compound a time after application. The corneum layer can therefore function in a dual capacity—as a barrier and as a reservoir, storing compounds for hours or perhaps days after application on the skin.

Some small compounds may preferentially pass into the skin through the pilosebaceous orifice and the sweat glands. For those compounds, differences in the density of hair follicles and sweat ducts in various body sites may also account for different rates of penetration.

Illness can change the rate of topical absorption. For example, diabetes is known to change the structure of epidermal membranes and capillary function, increasing the skin's absorption capabilities in chronic diabetics. In addition, chemical penetration varies on different parts of the body. On the face and scalp, for example, absorption is often five to ten times higher than elsewhere.

HOW PRODUCTS PENETRATE

The corneum layer, with its strongly and tightly bound cells, is the greatest obstacle to product penetration. The second barrier is the epidermal-dermal junction or basement membrane. If one skin function is to serve as a barrier, protecting the body from penetration by foreign matter, how is it that chemicals or cosmetic ingredients can penetrate? Structurally, the skin absorbs. This absorption takes place through the pilosebaceous pores, the ducts of the sweat glands, the intercellular channels that bind cells together, and the cellular system itself.

In reality, a large percentage of topically applied products never penetrate the corneum layer due to one or more of the following reasons:

- molecular size (too large)
- retention or binding on the surface by other ingredients present in the product
- evaporation (if volatile)

- adhesion to surface corneum cells and then loss by exfoliation

What does manage to penetrate can:

- permeate through the epidermal cells and cellular cement.
- form a reservoir by binding in the corneum layer (or in the subcutaneous fat) from which it may be very slowly released.
- be metabolized by the skin's own process.
- penetrate into the dermis and remain there.
- penetrate into the dermis and be absorbed into microcirculation by the capillaries. (This is an absorption method increasingly used in the pharmaceutical field. The nicotine patch is an example.)

The understanding of product penetration has greatly increased in the last few years. Certain products and ingredients can overcome the skin barrier via absorption. Yet, this action is dependent upon numerous factors including the ingredient(s), molecular size, other compounds present in the products, the duration the material is left on the skin, amount applied, condition of the skin, body temperature, and even the health of the individual.

Although the whys and hows of product penetration have been established, it is also important to look at what can affect this action.

Factors Affecting Product Penetration

The corneum layer's health is a major factor affecting the rate and extent of skin absorption. Another is skin hydration. One of the most common methods to increase penetration is through occlusion (trapping liquid or gas—in this case in the corneum) that prevents surface evaporation of water, which further increases corneum layer hydration. This is the concept behind the use of masks in skin care.

Environments with relative humidity greater than 80% may also result in significant skin hydration. It must be noted, however, that while the skin has great water absorption capabilities it does not have equally great water retention capabilities. As the corneum layer softens due to excessive hydration (as in the case of prolonged baths), its barrier function is weakened, allowing for increased moisture loss and dehydration.

When an individual's skin is exposed to high ambient temperatures or strenuous exercise, product absorption (depending on the product's composition) is believed to increase up to threefold, primarily as a result of increased blood flow. In this case, increased skin hydration or perspiration also aids absorption.

The primary path for a chemical's penetration of the corneum layer is through lipid-containing intercellular spaces. Therefore, the epidermal lipid composition affects permeation. Given the miscibility (ability to mix) of oil with oil, therapeutic chemicals dissolved in oil-based carriers will permeate more easily through the epidermal layers than those dissolved in water. The carriers in which therapeutic ingredients are dissolved or mixed for convenient application and control of ingredient concentration play a major role in determining the rate of penetration. In some instances, chemical absorption may be limited by the carrier used rather than by the barrier function of the skin layers.

Today, product penetration is undergoing a great deal of research in the scientific field. Though much is discussed, this knowledge is constantly being updated as new measuring techniques, insights on skin functioning, product interactions, and degrees of penetration are better understood. Let's not forget that until recently popular and scientific belief maintained that nothing penetrated the skin. Product penetration is now so thoroughly accepted that the new concern is the speed and depth of penetration rather than penetration itself.

PRODUCT TESTING

As a note to product penetration, a very common and reasonable question arises as to testing methods and exactly how scientists know that products work in a particular way.

Products are tested in vitro and in vivo, often using extensive and complex computer programs. For in vitro testing, skin is grown in glass containers where cells reproduce twenty times or more. Skin samples are also obtained from patients undergoing plastic surgery or some other type of surgery where a segment of skin is eliminated. Work in vitro presents great advantages in terms of time, lower cost, and ethical considerations when toxicity is a potential problem. Products tested in vivo are tested on living animals and human beings. In vivo studies provide the most direct, relevant, and conclusive information, especially when the systemic effect—how the body as a whole is affected— of a product is being questioned.

In the case of products that remain on the skin's surface or in the corneum layer, researchers apply the product on the skin and then remove the skin by stripping with adhesive tape or by scratching. The rate of product penetration and cellular change at different levels of penetration is then studied, usually through complex computer models.

For products believed to penetrate into the dermal layers, their systemic effect is also evaluated with sophisticated computer models that allow researchers to see not only how deep the product penetrated but what changes it caused in the cellular structure. The compounds under consideration are marked and their penetration is followed into the skin and the blood, urine, and other body fluids. However, the amounts penetrating the skin are frequently quite small and require extremely sensitive equipment to detect their presence in the body.

Before a product's massive introduction into the marketplace, premarket human testing has always been the ultimate test of a product's mildness and acceptability by consumers.

To answer our original product penetration questions, given what we now know about how the skin functions, products (or more accurately specific ingredients contained therein) can, under the right conditions, penetrate—generally via absorption. Penetration however may not be all important for product efficacy. In certain cases, it may actually be undesirable or counterproductive. A daytime protector, for example, should remain on the skin's surface forming a film or network to prevent moisture loss. When it comes to the need for penetration to actually treat a skin type or condition, there is a limit as to how far a cosmetic is "allowed" to penetrate before it falls out of the cosmetic category and into the pharmaceutical one.

Great progress is being made in cosmetic chemistry and in understanding how the skin works. With this knowledge, new product technologies increasingly appear able to facilitate product penetration, and with the proper ingredients there seems to be true enhancement of the skin.

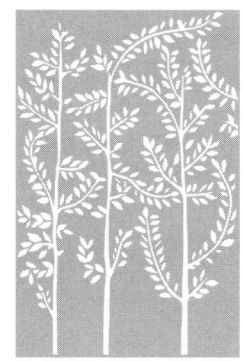

Chapter 3
SKIN TYPES AND
SKIN CONDITIONS

The correct identification of skin types and conditions is key for successfully selecting effective cosmetic products. Although there are as many subtle variations to skin types and conditions as there are human beings, certain prevalent characteristics allow us to group skin types into three classifications and skin conditions into another six. In most cases individuals have a combination of skin types plus one or more skin conditions. Products are generally formulated to address specific situations.

This chapter is designed to help relate skin requirements to the cosmetic ingredients most beneficial to an individual' s skin. It is also useful for identifying why a given product may or may not provide expected results and for identifying potential negative reactions.

SKIN TYPES

Skin types are hereditary and are the result of oil glands functioning. Skin types can be classified into three categories—normal, oily, and dry. In most cases, individuals have a combination of skin types such as an oily T-zone (around eyes and nose) and normal cheeks. Of course, these skin types occur in varying degrees, such as very oily or very dry, slightly oily or slightly dry.

The notion that one person's skin can be oily and dry is more commonly a confusion in concept than a reality. For example, when people describe the skin as having been oily and all of a sudden being dry, they are referring to an oily skin type that is losing moisture because of overdrying. This is usually caused by excessive use of astringents, soaps, and/or scrubs in an attempt to reduce the amount of oil secretion. While the skin is an oily type, this dryness should be considered a skin condition and is properly referred to as dehydration—a lack of water moisture rather than oil.

In general, there seems to be such an obsession with oiliness that people forget about moisture. To hear "I don't need a moisturizer, my skin is oily" is quite common. It is important to remember that the skin has oil and water, and that **both** are important for its beauty and retarding the aging process.

Normal Skin

Normal skin has perfect hydration, muscle tone, and resilience produced by moisture and the adipose tissues. There is strong biological activity at the basal layer, blood circulation is active, and the metabolism is balanced. Normal skin looks soft, moist, plump, and dewy and has a healthy glow and color. The corneum layer shows a fine texture, and there are no visible wrinkles, fine lines, or open pores.

The best example of normal skin is that of children, from birth usually until puberty. Oil glands functioning at a normal rate of secretion are also seen in mature individuals who once had oily skin. With age, the rate of oil gland secretion slows down and becomes normal. However, the normal skin found in this second case varies from the normal skin of youth insofar as there is no strong biological activity at the basal layer and, in most cases, suppleness and color have deteriorated.

Aging is the primary factor that deteriorates normal skin. Other factors include insufficient water intake and an inadequate diet. Tea, coffee, and sodas do not make up for water as the body processes them differently. Food devoid of vitamins, enzymes, and amino acids does not provide the cells with the nourishment necessary for cellular reproduction and growth. Improper skin care such as lack of cleansing is quite prevalent in children and teenagers due to the lack of skin care awareness. The use of harsh soaps and scrubs, climate, and environment contribute to the deterioration of normal skin. Sun exposure and exposure to the elements without protection dries, dehydrates, and ages the skin.

Normal skin requires proper cleansing, morning and evening. The consistent use of protective moisturizers during the day to prevent moisture loss and hydrating creams at night is essential. An occasional exfoliation is also beneficial. Sun protection is extremely important, even for children. Children should not be allowed on the beach without a proper sunscreen or in the snow without a good protective cream.

Oily Skin

Oily skin is a hereditary condition that develops due to overactive sebaceous glands. This activity is controlled by the androgen, or masculine, hormone. Oily skin can be recognized by its shiny, thick, and firm appearance. Pores look enlarged, usually due to oil entrapped in the pilosebaceous follicle. Enlarged pores become aggravated with a dehydrated condition. An oily complexion tends to look dirty and neglected, occasionally with blemishes on the chin or the forehead area, and feels oily to the touch.

Hot and humid climates tend to exacerbate oil gland secretion making the skin more oily. Oily skin problems can be aggravated by the misuse of skin care products and the tendency to dry the skin either through the use of harsh soaps or the excessive use of astringents or scrubs. Overstimulation of skin functions through scrubbing or stimulating massage should be avoided.

Exfoliating products, such as alpha hydroxyacids (AHAs) and exfoliating enzymes, help improve the look and texture of oily skin. Products with active substances, including botanicals, that may help regulate or reduce oil gland secretions are also appropriate. These could include, but are not limited to, royal jelly, vitamin F, and rosemary. Mint and thyme act as solvents on the fats with an added action on the sebaceous glands.

Care requires thorough yet gentle cleansing morning and evening. Daytime protective moisturizers will help the skin maintain its suppleness and moisture. Evening creams should help regulate oil gland secretion. It is most important to keep oily skin clean and hydrated with appropriate cleansing and care. AHA exfoliators and weekly use of enzyme peels is highly recommended. When properly cared for, this is the preferred skin type since it delays the wrinkle process.

Dry Skin

Dry skin develops as a result of sebaceous gland underactivity. Skin dryness, though hereditary like skin oiliness, also results from the aging process. As all body activities slow down, oil gland activity slows as well. Dry skin tends to be dehydrated. Its lack of oil diminishes its ability to retain moisture since oil in the skin acts as a natural barrier against moisture loss. Dry skin is characterized as very fine, overly delicate, and thin. Lack of sufficient oil secretion deprives the skin of sufficient "glue" to retain cells in the corneum layer. As a result, dry skin has fewer cells in the corneum layer than oily skin. In dry skin, pores are almost invisible. The skin also tends to wrinkle easily and is often filled with tiny superficial lines.

Dry skin problems are aggravated by exposure to the sun, wind, and heat. Improper skin care, such as excessive lubrication and lack of protection against moisture loss especially during the day, further exacerbates this problem.

Care for dry skin should include daytime protection using products containing sealants such as silicone or collagen-based products. These products form a layer on the surface of the skin and reduce moisture loss. In addition, a program of good skin nourishment and lubrication with appropriate night creams is highly recommended. The use of nourishing, hydrating masks is also advisable for dry skin. Appropriate ingredients for dry skin can include, but are not limited to, vitamin E (usually listed as tocopherol), Ajidew, ginseng, dandelion extract, avocado oil, macadamia nut oil, and some of the newest ingredients such as hyaluronic acid, ceramides, and mucopolysaccharides.

SKIN CONDITIONS

Skin conditions develop over time and can apply to all three skin types (with the exception of acne, which is not usually found in combination with dry skin), leading to the many combinations that make everyone's skin unique. The most common skin conditions are dehydration, couperose, sensitivity, pigmentation, aging, and acne vulgaris.

Dehydration

This is one of the most common skin conditions. It means a lack of sufficient moisture in the cellular system and intercellular channels. Dehydrated skin looks dry, scaly, and flaky. It feels tight. When gently pulled, the skin "crinkles," similar to pulling a corner of very thin tissue paper. Sometimes the skin appears as if it had an additional thin layer of skin placed on top. This would be particularly evident on the nose and forehead.

Dehydration is caused by excessive perspiration, lack of sufficient sebum to prevent evaporation of natural moisture, poor metabolism, and/or insufficient water intake. Dehydration is aggravated by atmospheric conditions including too much sun and wind; not using sunscreens and/or daytime protective moisturizers; using inappropriate skin care products; cleansing with harsh soaps and water; drinking tea, coffee, soda, or diuretics; and not drinking enough water.

Dehydration is one of the most difficult skin conditions to diagnose. It is usually confused with dryness, technically a lack of oil. Unfortunately they have many similarities. Both dry and oily skin types may be dehydrated. Dry skin can be dehydrated because thin skin has difficulty in retaining inner moisture. Oily skin becomes dehydrated through the use of harsh soaps and the excessive use of astringents. When oily skin becomes dehydrated the surface layers of cells harden up and block oil secretion. The result is an entrapment of the oils under the corneum layer. This is particularly detrimental in the case of someone with acne as it results also in the entrapment of the infection. To end the confusion the best approach is to first diagnose the skin type and then the skin condition.

Care for dehydrated skin should include daytime protective moisturizers. These help seal the natural moisture of the skin and reduce moisture loss. Masks ought to be applied on a weekly or biweekly basis depending on the level of dehydration. Products with hydrating ingredients are ideal for this skin condition.

Couperose

Couperose is temporary or chronic redness appearing on the face. It appears as small, dilated, winding, bright red blood vessels on cheeks, around the nose, and sometimes on the chin.

Couperose occurs primarily as a result of poor elasticity in the capillarian wall. When there is a sudden rush of blood because of blushing, excessive heat, or other stimuli, the capillaries expand, making room for the increase of blood. When the amount of blood recedes, the capillaries contract to their normal size. If the capillarian wall is not sufficiently elastic, it will expand but may not contract again to its original shape or size. The result is a distended capillary that will hold blood cells within its structure thus giving the appearance of diffuse or local redness.

Couperose is aggravated by atmospheric agents such as hot climates, by the use of excessively cold or hot water, nervous disorders, digestive disorders, saunas, exercise that causes the face to turn very red, drinking very hot liquids, eating spicy foods, and blushing. If using Retin-A^{TM}, consult with a physician as it may aggravate the couperose condition as well.

Care should be taken that skins with this condition are not exposed to excessively hot or cold water. Night creams or lotions that help strengthen the capillarian walls are helpful.

Products with soothing, and vasoconstrictive ingredients are also beneficial.

Sensitivity

While sensitivity can apply to couperose skin, many times it is the result of an isolated condition. It affects dry and oily skin types and is difficult to diagnose. The causes of sensitivity are not clear. The pilosebaceous orifice is not a tube like the sweat gland, but rather an invagination (folding of outer layer to form an inner layer) of the skin. The hair follicle is surrounded by a very delicate membrane separating a layer of mucosum cells from the hair follicle. When products penetrate through this follicle, if the separating membrane and the mucosum cells are very delicate they could easily be irritated by chemicals. Other reasons, primarily seen in dry skins, are a very uneven, scaly, or thin corneum layer, allowing for the penetration of products into the more delicate epidermal layer.

A sensitive skin reaction can express itself as redness, itching, burning, and in the worst of cases as small pustules sometimes filled with a watery liquid. In this last case it is best to refer to a dermatologist.

Skin sensitivity is usually aggravated by particular ingredients. Certain preservative ingredients are known to be sensitizing. In other instances plant pollen can be enough of a factor to cause an unpleasant reaction in sensitive skin. Facial scrubbing and the use of astringents with a high level of alcohol will definitely aggravate this skin condition. People with sensitive skin should use very gentle and delicate products. Cosmetic formulations with added botanicals that have antiallergenic, soothing, and healing properties are helpful, and anti-inflammatory agents are also beneficial.

Pigmentation

Pigmentation problems result from an uneven distribution of melanin over the skin surface either due to pigment accumulation as in the case of actinic keratosis and lentigo, or because of uneven melanin production by the melanocytes, as in the case of melasma.

Melanin is produced by the melanocyte cell located in the germinative layer of the epidermis. After its formation and as it matures, the melanocyte transforms itself into melanosoma. The melanosoma, as it matures and continues its movement from the germinative to the corneum layer transforms itself into melanin. Melanin acts as a filter, protecting the skin and body against the harmful effects of the sun's radiation. The irritation on the skin's surface caused by sun exposure translates itself into a greater production of melanin. A suntan is basically the body's protective response against internal skin damage. The amount of melanin that reaches the epidermis gives the skin its color.

Lentigo, commonly known as age spots, occurs when there is an uneven accumulation of melanin deposits in the epidermal surface layers. In the case of melasma, or local hyperpigmentation, the pigmentation results when the melanocytes produce a greater amount of melanin in a given area of the skin, and/or when the melanin is not properly absorbed by the keratinic cells. Melasma occurs as a result of hormonal imbalances caused by pregnancy, the use of birth control pills, menopause, or nervous disorders. Dark spots can also be the result of surface irritation of the skin as those caused by acne conditions.

The best treatment for pigmentation is based on bleaching agents and the attempt to regulate melanocyte activity. The bleaching agents can include hydroquinone, kojic acid, linden, and yarrow. Some bleaching agents should only be applied at night as some of the ingredients tend to react with sunlight and further aggravate the problem. In all cases when using a bleaching agent the use of sunscreens during the day is mandatory to attain best results and to avoid the negative irritating effect of the sun. Failure to use a sunscreen could neutralize whatever result the bleaching product may give.

Aging

Aging skin can be recognized by its poor elasticity, flaccidity (lack of normal firmness), and sagging due to the loosening of the fibroblast in the dermis; the accentuation of lines and wrinkles as a result of increased dryness; and dehydration caused by skin thinning and the decrease of oil gland activity. The complexion looks withered and takes on an "old ivory" shade as the production of melanin diminishes.

Skin aging is connected to a deficiency of nutritional components in the different tissues, cellular destruction through excessive sun exposure, the effect of free radicals on the cellular membrane, and a deterioration in the genetic programming of the DNA. All this brings about the atrophy of the skin and consequently a general process of degeneration. Aging skin results from the passage of time, overexposure to the sun that destroys cellular ability to reproduce, lack of proper care while young, health problems, and hormonal imbalances. Additional causes are improper nutrition, thereby not providing appropriate nourishment to the epidermis for cellular reproduction and growth, stress, and lifestyle.

The treatment for aging skin should emphasize hydration. Moisture in the skin and the intercellular channels is key to youthful looking skin. Products offering protection such as protective moisturizers and sunblocks are recommended at all times. Stimulating, hydrating, and revitalizing active ingredients are very important for mature skin, especially in products for night use. Weekly use of masks will aid in the hydration process. The regular use of specialty ampules with stimulating and revitalizing active ingredients will also prove very helpful.

Acne Vulgaris

This acne condition is recognized by infection spots and pustules. They could be numerous or sparse, but they will be small. Skin with acne vulgaris will be oily, and in many cases it may look dirty and improperly cared for and have blackheads, whiteheads, and clogged pores. Acne is not an internal disease surfacing on the skin, but rather the combined result of four elements—the androgen hormones, excessive cellular keratinization and agglomeration in the corneum layer and the sebaceous follicle, oil production, and an overpopulation of a bacteria known as the

Propionibacterium acnes (P. acnes). Other types of acne, such as cystic and rosacea, should be referred to a dermatologist and care be given under medical supervision.

Some of the many factors said to aggravate acne include excessive oiliness, improper skin care preventing the thorough removal of oil and dirt from the skin, hormonal imbalances, hyperkeratinization, food allergies and sensitivities, lack of vitamins (especially vitamin A), and insufficient acidity in the skin (the skin's pH is believed to control bacteria population) Acne is also aggravated by climatic conditions, especially heat and humidity, which increase bacteria development; the use of astringents and drying cosmetics; improper diet; stress; and picking.

Those with acne should emphasize cleansing at home and by a skin care professional and skin hydration. The most effective products are those with ingredients that regulate oil gland secretion, hydrate, heal, balance the pH of the skin, soothe, and reduce inflammation.

In diagnosing the skin it is recommended to **first identify skin type.** This will avoid confusing dryness (lack of oil) with dehydration (lack of water). It will also greatly assist in the proper identification of a skin care product with ingredients of most benefit to the skin in question. Proper diagnosis of a skin type and/or condition is key to identifying the correct skin care product with the most valuable therapeutic ingredients.

Chapter 4
DEFINITION
OF TERMS

acid—used in cosmetic formulations to neutralize substances that otherwise would be too alkaline. Acids are also employed as exfoliating and peeling agents (e.g., alpha hydroxyacids). Other compounds referred to as acids are active principles that perform a specific function based on their own particular properties (e.g., hyaluronic acid). Cosmetics with a very low acid level will be irritating to the skin. An acid is technically defined as a proton donor (*see* atom). The term *acid* refers to the pH level of a substance ranging from 0 for the most acidic substance to 6.9 for the least acidic.

active principle (AKA active ingredient)—an ingredient with "treatment value." When placed on the skin it would perform a therapeutic or beneficial function such as healing, hydrating, soothing, toning, etc.

Chapter 4

alcohols—widely used in cosmetics as solvents, carriers, and astringents. When used as active ingredients they are considered antiseptic, antiviral, and bactericidal. Alcohols are organic compounds containing a hydroxyl group (OH) in their molecule. They are recognized by the suffix *-ol* such as ethanol for ethyl alcohol; isopropanol for isopropyl alcohol; and in essential oils such as geraniol, nerol, and linalol. Compounds listed with an *-ol* ending should therefore be recognized as alcohols even if the word "alcohol" does not follow.

aldehyde—can be used as a chemical reagent, solvent, fragrance, or, when used as an active ingredient, as a soothing or antiseptic compound. An aldehyde is an organic compound containing a carboxyl group (O and H) in its molecule. This is different from the OH of the alcohols. In an aldehyde the "O" for oxygen and the "H" for hydrogen are each individually attached to the "C" carbon atom. In the alcohol group the "OH" is attached as a unit. Aldehydes are generally recognized by the suffix *-al*, such as citral, geranial, or ethanal for ethyl aldehyde.

$$\begin{array}{cc} \text{H} & \\ | & \\ \text{C}{=}\text{O} & \qquad \text{C}{-}\text{OH} \\ \text{aldehyde} & \qquad \text{alcohol} \end{array}$$

alkaline—used in cosmetics usually to balance formulas with an undesired acid level. An alkaline is defined as a proton acceptor (*see* atom). It is a pH level measurement; a substance of 7.1 is the least alkaline and a substance of 14 is the most alkaline. Cosmetics with a high alkaline level will be irritating to the skin.

antioxidant—the definition refers to a compound that prevents other compounds from oxidizing (such as rusting) or becoming rancid (as in the case of fats and oils). Today this also refers to an ingredient's ability to counteract free radical activity in antiaging cosmetics.

aromatherapy—refers to the use of essential oils for therapeutic purposes and perfumery. Its use in skin care ranges from a marketing tool to the fragrancing of cosmetics to the therapeutic value associated with the topical applications of essential oils. This includes topical use as well as more subtle psychological changes resulting from scent inhalation, including an overall feeling of well-being, mood changes, and even an increase and/or decrease in productivity levels.

astringent—refers to the constriction of tissues and the resulting improvement in the appearance of skin with large, open pores. An astringent is also used to reduce the oil content on the skin's surface. Excessive use of astringents may result in surface dryness.

atom—the smallest component of an element still retaining the element's properties. An atom is composed of positive and negative charges called protons and electrons respectively. The protons are in the nucleus of the atom and the electrons are found in layers around the nucleus. Each atom has the same number of electrons and protons. A combination of atoms forms a larger substance called a molecule.

bioavailable (AKA bioactive; bioavailability)—refers to the ingredient(s) or amount of ingredient(s) available for the skin's use given formulation and skin characteristics.

botanical—a plant extract containing active plant constituents that can elicit certain biological responses when applied on the skin. A reference to botanicals may imply use in a variety of forms. It could indicate the use of a complete plant extract containing the same phytocomplex, or combination of natural components present in the plant, or a combination of particular elements such as flavonoids and terpenes. It could also indicate the use of pure elements isolated from the plant. Biological responses obtained from the use of botanicals are often associated with the concentration level of the active constituents present in the formulation, the skin's capability to absorb these, the effect that other ingredients present in the formulation might have on the active constituent, and its degree of penetration.

Although botanicals were used by ancient societies as remedies for a variety of external and internal disorders, the measured and tested effectiveness of synthetic ingredients nearly reduced their value to pure folklore and hearsay. Today, however, scientists are discovering the individual chemical constituents responsible for the therapeutic virtues long attributed to these botanicals. Such is the case, for example, of balm mint and licorice. In the case of other botanicals, no scientific data exists to explain their therapeutic behavior. Yet, trial and observation are leading to research that will validate visual data indicating therapeutic value and perhaps therapeutic constituents. The general belief is that when botanicals are used in low concentrations their primary value may be for marketing and product labeling purposes rather than true therapeutic effect. As skin care product labeling regulations do not require percentage disclosure, the value of botanical use in cosmetic formulations remains clouded by skepticism.

buffered—refers to a chemical process by which a compound(s) is added to a formulation in order to keep the formulation's pH unchanged regardless of what else is added into it.

carbomers—a group of high-molecular-weight polymers widely used as thickeners, suspending agents, and emulsion stabilizers for a variety of skin care products. The high clarity and unique texture they impart have led the way in the evolution of the gel product form. The benefits associated with carbomers include specific texture and formulation flow control, highly effective oil/water emulsion stabilization, and permanent suspension of insoluble or immiscible ingredients.

carrier (AKA vehicle)—This product component may have a great influence on a formulation's active principle(s) as it may affect the active's efficacy, stability, and time release, as well as skin tolerance and final location in the different skin levels. A carrier can also determine the ease of product application.

chemical reaction—refers to the transformation of one or more substances into one or more different substances.

color—can be found listed as FD&C, D&C, and Ext. D&C. FD&C colors are approved for use in food, drugs, and cosmetics. D&C colors may be used only in drugs and cosmetics, including those that come in contact with mucous membranes and those that are ingested. An Ext. D&C listing indicates the use of a color certified for use in drugs and cosmetics that do not come in contact with mucous membranes and that are not ingested. (**NOTE:** these definitions should be used only as guidelines, as some FD&C colors are no longer approved for cosmetic use.)

A color listing can be broken down into three parts. For example, with FD&C Red No. 4 the first part indicates under which category of FDA certification the pigment falls (here it is an FD&C), the second gives the color (Red), and the number indicates which red is being used. If listed as FD&C Yellow No. 6 Al Lake, the Al Lake refers to "aluminum lake" and indicates the use of an organic pigment of the lake group—a water-soluble dye absorbed on alumina.

Three types of coloring matter are used in cosmetic products—inorganic, organic, and dyestuffs. Inorganic pigments are insoluble compounds based on metal ions, tend to have good stability, and are widely used in eye and face makeup. Organic pigments tend to be bright but offer less variety in shades. This type of pigment is further divided into three subsets—lakes (water-soluble dyes absorbed on alumina), toners (organic barium or calcium salts), and true pigments. Although the true pigments are the least popular for use in cosmetics, they are the most stable of the three. The lakes are the least stable, and toners fall in between. Dyestuffs are used primarily in toiletry products such as shampoos and lotions. There are six classes of water-soluble dyestuffs commonly used in cosmetics and whose stability is dependent on chemical structure. These include azo, indigoid, and xanthene.

Since the creation of FDA regulations on colors, the types of colors certified as safe and appropriate for use in food, drugs, and cosmetics has gone from 116 permitted in 1959 to 35 permitted in 1988. The colors listed on an ingredient label fall under FDA jurisdiction.

comedogenic—used to describe an ingredient that tends to increase keratinocyte agglomeration in the pilosebaceous follicle, thus creating a blockage of the follicle and causing the formation of comedones.

controlled release—a term used to describe a particular way an active ingredient is made available to the skin. The term encompasses systems based on encapsulating technologies such as liposomes or polymer entrapment. The concept of controlled release is to provide continuous and systematic delivery of the active ingredient(s), thereby avoiding the "peak and valley" of availability characteristically associated with regular topical applications. Encapsulated or entrapped actives can have a more controlled evaporation and greater skin compatibility, cause less irritation, and maximize the amount of time an active ingredient (e.g., a moisturizer or a sunscreen) is present on the skin surface or within the epidermis. When required, such a system will reduce potential penetration. These systems can release their content, usually at once, by breakage due to pressure, abrasion, or dissolution of their shell. *See also* encapsulation.

cosmeceutical—a combination of the words *cosmetic* and *pharmaceutical*. This term has been coined to describe cosmetic preparations with biological claims. Some describe them as cosmetic drugs that include antiaging creams, antiwrinkle lotions, and similar products. There is the belief that these products, though marketed as cosmetics, could have drug claims and hence ought to be treated as a separate category of product, one that should undergo premarket testing for clearance. From the regulatory standpoint cosmeceuticals are in a gray area and are under further government scrutiny. From the commercial standpoint the term *cosmeceuticals* is being used to indicate that a given product may have greater efficacy than whatever can be said under cosmetic claims.

delivery system—refers to the means by which an active principle is delivered to the site of action in the skin. Delivery systems can affect skin reaction, ingredient penetration, and even ingredient efficacy.

emollient—often termed skin conditioners, emollients are fatty substances with lubricating action that make the skin feel softer and more pliable. Emollients also have a hydrating effect by reducing moisture evaporation from the skin surface via water diffusion into the corneum layer and underlying tissues. Although virtually any fatty material can make the skin feel softer, different emollients produce different results and skin feel. There are over 600 emollients providing a variety of characteristics to a formulation—oily, dry, draggy, slippery, penetrating, nonpenetrating, shiny, dull, or any combination the formulator wishes to achieve. The selection of an emollient is a formulator's choice based on desired product performance and the other ingredients present in the formulation.

emulsion—oil and water blended together as one substance, such as a cream or a lotion, by use of an emulsifier.

emulsifier—in a homogenized system, holds the oil-based and water-based ingredients together, thereby avoiding their separation in the cosmetic formulation.

encapsulation (AKA microencapsulation)—the process of enveloping microscopic amounts of substance in a thin film of polymer. Liposomes are an example of encapsulation. Some of the many reasons for the use of encapsulation in cosmetic formulations are controlled release, reduction of irritation, and reduction of evaporation. *See also* controlled release.

enzyme—a biological catalyst of vegetable or animal origin that is able to accelerate or produce a chemical change. The most common enzymes are those of vegetable origin, such as papain from papaya. Enzymes are generally used as exfoliants or peels. The correct concentration in a formulation is of great importance—too little will not be effective, too much may cause adverse reactions or could even be toxic. Presently, enzymes like superoxide dismutase (SOD) may be among the most firmly established of free radical reducing enzymes.

essential fatty acid (EFA)—form the basic building blocks of body fats and cellular membranes. Since cell membranes are largely made of phospholipids, topically applied EFAs may be metabolized in the skin, normalizing the cell lipid layer and improving the water retention capability of the corneum layer.

essential oil—a volatile oily substance produced by many plants. Essential oils contain vitamins, hormones, antibiotics, and/or antiseptics. These oils are present as tiny droplets between the plant's cells. They play an important role in the plant's biochemistry, and are also responsible for its fragrance. Essential oils have many established and attributed properties, including antiseptic, antibiotic, soothing, and calming. These oils are extracted by a variety of methods that allow the integrity of the oil to be maintained. Distillation is the most common method. The yield of essential oils varies between 0.005% and 10% of the plant depending on the type of plant. The lower the yield, the more expensive the essential oil. The quality and chemistry of essential oils may vary according to the part of the plant from which the oil was extracted (root, bark, flowers, leaf), the time of day and/or year in which it was picked, the location where the plant grows (lowlands, highlands), and the methods of cultivation.

esters—products resulting from the combination of organic acids and alcohols. They can be natural or synthetic and liquid or solid depending on properties of the reacting substances. Being insoluble in water, they replace oils and fats to provide a more uniform composition and preservation. They have good skin tolerance and a lubricating and emollient action.

Esters are also found in essential oils. Often even small amounts of characteristic esters are crucial for the finer notes in the fragrance of an essential oil.

fatty acid—*see* essential fatty acid.

flavonoids—considered active substances extracted from plants and capable of acting as free radical scavengers.

fragrance—natural and synthetic fragrances are added to a cosmetic formulation to make the product smell better. Today, fragrances are added to achieve subtly communicated messages such as image, market positioning, and even performance. Studies conducted on consumer perception of product efficacy clearly demonstrated that, using the same product base, consumers gave the product a different performance rating depending on the fragrance used.

Fragrances have also been the source of cosmetic allergies. An FDA study determined that more than 1% of all cosmetic allergic contact dermatitis cases were due to fragrances. Observations indicate that in reality this percentage may be significantly higher—7% to 18% of all individuals may have some form of sensitivity or intolerance to fragrances. As a result, products positioned as hypoallergenic are fragranceless.

On an ingredient label, perhaps one of the only certain ways to know if a product was purposely fragranced is with a listing of "Fragrance" alone or followed by a number (e.g., Fragrance No. 012345). This, however, should not be taken as an indication of a synthetic fragrance. It indicates the use of a particular fragrance or fragrance mix. Terminology such as "plant extracts" indicates extracts used for therapeutic purposes and/or fragrancing; there is no definite way of knowing by just looking at the label.

With the increased popularity of aromatherapy, many skin care products, particularly salon treatment lines, depend on already incorporated botanicals for fragrance. This is appealing based on the dual functioning of botanicals or botanical mixes. Not only does the formulator achieve potential therapeutic value but he or she is able to add fragrance without offending a consumer's sense of "green" or creating a fear of increasing skin sensitivity.

free radicals (AKA reactive oxygen species)—atoms or molecules with an unpaired electron. They are unstable, highly reactive, and are produced in the skin by Ultraviolet (UV) light, heat, and radiation. Free radicals can severely damage the skin by attacking cellular membranes.

free radical scavengers (AKA anti-free radicals, antioxidants)—components that counteract the destructive effect of free radical activity. Compounds such as vitamin E, the different tocopherols, vitamin C, ascorbic acid, and the flavonoids are examples of ingredients currently considered free radical scavengers. They can be systemically or topically incorporated to help reduce the free radical effect by decomposing the free radicals into compounds against which the body has defenses.

humectant—used in cosmetic formulations to increase the skin's moisture content. Humectants have the ability to bind moisture and are considered moisturizers.

hydrolysis—a chemical process by which complex proteins are degraded to smaller molecules of lower molecular weight, including into their individual amino acid components. Hydrolysis can be performed via acid reactions or enzymatic action. Hydrolyzed proteins, therefore, are proteins of lower molecular weight than their source and have greater skin affinity. Hence, they are more easily incorporated into cosmetic formulations. Generally, the term hydrolyzed, so commonly found on cosmetic labels, does not identify the amino acids involved nor the process of hydrolysis used.

hygroscopic—used to describe an ingredient that readily absorbs and retains moisture.

hypoallergenic—used to described a cosmetic product as one that does not produce allergic reactions. The causes and varieties of allergies are so broad and widespread that it is very difficult to state that a product is truly hypoallergenic. Allergenicity is not a matter of the product but rather the sensitivity of the individual. Usually this term is applied to products that are fragrance free and have a select type of preservative. Products with essential oils and plant extracts pose a greater risk of allergic reactions.

liquid crystals—described primarily as compounds that can encapsulate active substances and allow for a time-release pattern. They are a recent development and are considered intermediates between solids and liquids.

lipid—constitutes, by weight, 6–10% of the normal corneum layer. Lipids are important for the corneum layer's healthy structure and function. They are found primarily in the intercellular spaces, accounting for a significant volume of the corneum layer. These intercellular lipids provide a barrier to the passage of a variety of substances through the skin.

Lipids incorporated into cosmetics help moisturize the skin by renewing its barrier function, either by replacing lipids that have been removed with washing, allowing epidermal lipids to remain despite adverse environments, or renewing the skin's ability to bind moisture.

The skin's barrier function against moisture loss is proportional to the lipid content within the corneum layer.

molecule—a substance made from a combination of similar or different atoms. Molecules have their own characteristic set of properties. For example, a water molecule is composed of two hydrogen atoms and one oxygen atom. The size of a molecule is established by its number of atoms and will determine the compound's ability to penetrate the skin layers. The larger a molecule, the less its ability to penetrate the skin. In addition, the larger the molecule the lower its ability to evaporate and diffuse through the skin. Smaller molecules have greater volatility (evaporation ability).

natural moisturizing factor (NMF)—found in the corneum layer, the NMF is comprised of hygroscopic, water-soluble substances that regulate the layer's selective permeability. The NMF is composed of about 40% free amino acids, 12% PCA, 12% lactose, 7% urea, and approximately 30% of a large variety of other materials. Exposure to harsh detergents and climatic conditions can result in decreased NMF levels, rendering the skin fragile and dry.

The design of modern moisturizers has depended on selecting various hygroscopic ingredients with properties and effects similar to the NMF and combining them with effective vehicles.

neutralized—when a chemical product has been added to bring the formulation's pH to near 7, or neutral. Partially neutralized is when a chemical product is added to move the compound pH toward 7 or a more neutral value.

oligoelement—refers to trace elements, such as zinc, copper, magnesium, or selenium, with important catalytic action in enzymatic reactions to ensure normal cell metabolism. Zinc salts, for example, have been found to aid in the faster absorption of drugs. When topically applied via a cosmetic preparation, the effect of oligoelements on the skin is not clearly established.

Some sources indicate that indiscriminate application of these elements, whether single or combined, may be absolutely ineffective and may even harm the skin. Others state that experimental tests indicate the presence of selected oligoelements in a formulation may improve a protein derivative's affinity for a moisturizing capacity.

pH—refers to the level of acidity or alkalinity of a given chemical ingredient or product. As the hydrogen in a substance determines the ingredient's or product's level of acidity or alkalinity, the symbol *pH* stands for the power (p) of the hydrogen molecule (H). The pH of acids ranges between 0 and 6.9 and of alkalines between 7.1 and 14. A pH of 7 is considered neutral.

phytotherapy—used to describe very dissimilar groups of processes and methods that use all or part of a plant for esthetics treatments. It includes the use of plant extracts, distilled waters, and essential oils.

Chapter 4

polyethylene glycol (PEG)—PEGs are compatible with a wide range of ingredients and are blended into a formulation to obtain the desired humectancy, viscosity, or melting point. PEGs make excellent solvents, binders, vehicles, humectants, lubricants, and bases. When they are listed with another ingredient (e.g., PEG 5 Stearate), it means that a polyethylene glycol (PEG) chain has been added to the ingredient to enhance water solubility. The numbers that follow any PEG listing indicate how many moles of PEG are contained. For example, PEG 5 Stearate means the polyethylene glycol ester of stearic acid containing 5 moles of polyethylene glycol.

polymers—part of the encapsulation concept used for the controlled release effect. They allow for the encapsulation of the active ingredient(s) and its controlled and sustained release. Polymers improve the delivery of lubricants and skin protectants and the duration of skin moisturization. They also act as emulsifiers. (*See also* controlled release.)

precipitate—small particles (above 1 micron) that have settled out of a suspension due to gravity or as a result of electrical discharge.

precursors—intermediate compounds of high biological potential that, when activated, are converted to another specific substance. This is the case, for example, of ergosterol (provitamin D_2) that is changed by ultraviolet radiation to vitamin D. Carotene (provitamin A) is a precursor that can be transformed into vitamin A.

Biological precursors are also defined as small molecules capable of penetrating the skin. A further precursor action is to become involved in the skin's biochemical process. This would allow for the conversion of the precursor into another compound(s) that could not penetrate if introduced in its regular state either because of molecular size or affinity problems. In this way, the compound is able to take part in the metabolic process of the skin.

Some substances labeled as biological precursors are said to stimulate the synthesis of collagen, elastin, proteoglycans, and structural glycoproteins.

preservative—added to cosmetic formulations for a variety of purposes including maintaining product integrity during consumer use as many undesirable microorganisms (usually seen as mold growth) may become a possible health hazard to the consumer; extending the shelf life of a product since cosmetic products are not refrigerated; preventing microbial growth that may occur during manufacturing and packaging.

An ideal preservative should include a broad antibacterial/antifungal spectrum; a lack of toxicity, irritating, or sensitizing effects; compatibiliity with other products in the formulation; compatibility with packaging.

Often companies use the term *preservative free* in cosmetics more as a marketing tool. Scientists believe that preservatives serve a very useful function in keeping cosmetics safe. The idea that preservative free cosmetics are safer than those with preservatives, especially products with a high bioactive ingredient content easily subject to bacterial growth at room temperature, is not necessarily true.

retinoids—substances belonging to the vitamin A group. Though they have the same molecular construction, they differ in molecular modifications, which changes their functional properties.

sensitizer—refers to an ingredient(s) that can provoke a sensitivity reaction on the skin such as redness, swelling, itching, or any other adverse reaction.

solubilizer—helps dissolve normally insoluble materials such as fragrances and oils.

surfactant (AKA surface active agents)—includes emulsifiers, foaming agents, solubilizers, wetting agents, and cleansers.

Foaming and cleansing agents are basic constituents of shampoos and cleansers. Emulsifiers are used in the preparation of creams and lotions. Solubilizers allow for incompatible ingredients to become part of a homogeneous solution. Wetting agents are needed to work with fine particle powders in preparing liquids and pastes. The present work in the cosmetic field is to develop low irritation surfactants that achieve a maximum emulsifying, solubilizing, and dispersing effect while causing minimal reaction with epidermal cells. Damaging effects of surfactants on skin manifest themselves as dryness, roughness, scaling, and redness. There are almost 2,000 different surfactants available to the cosmetic formulator.

Irritation by surfactants accounts for a large number of adverse skin reactions. The level of irritation depends on the type of surfactant used, its concentration, and duration of the contact with the skin. Exaggerated use of surfactants coupled with preexisting sensitivity; extremes of temperature or pH; low humidity; or co-use of other potential irritants such as abrasives, bleaches, or lipid solvents can bring about reactions such as skin irritation, inflammation, chapping, and roughness.

sunscreen—technically refers to chemicals and more loosely to entire formulations designed to protect the skin from harmful UV rays. Ideally, sunscreens should absorb both UVA and UVB rays. Yet, this could require the use of more than one absorber, since those effective against UVB do not necessarily work against UVA. There are 21 FDA approved sunscreen chemicals available to the product formulator.

As consumer awareness creates demand for products offering more protection and current market preferences dictate that some chemicals, popular in the past, not be employed (e.g., PABA), formulators are challenged to combine or create protection-offering alternatives. Achieving a higher sun protection factor (SPF) product is not necessarily a question of dropping in some more sunscreen chemicals. This may do the trick, but it can also increase the cost and irritancy of the finished product. Alternatives are necessary. One includes the incorporation of film formers and waterproofing agents such as tricontanyl PVP and polyquaternium-24 to assist obtaining uniformity and waterresistance upon product application. A second, becoming increasingly popular, is the use of UV reflectors such as titanium dioxide and zinc oxide. Both titanium dioxide and zinc oxide must undergo processes of refinement in order to make them cosmetically acceptable.

As sunscreen products gain in popularity, techniques for elegant and effective sun product formulation promise to continue meeting market demand.

sun protection factor (SPF)—the amount of ultraviolet energy required to produce a minimal redness on unprotected skin. It refers to UVB protection.

thickening/gelling agents—provide "body" to cosmetics, increase their stability, improve suspending action, and contribute to application and feel. Some have film-forming characteristics, impart skin affinity, and can act as carriers/releasers for active ingredients. Most of these agents used by cosmetic formulators are synthetic. Only some 10% are of natural origin.

ultraviolet radiation—invisible ultraviolet light irradiated by the sun that varies in wavelengths. These wavelengths are known as UVA, which penetrates deeply into the skin causing a phototoxic effect at the dermal level, and UVB, a shorter wavelength whose penetration and concentration are almost exclusively in the epidermal layer causing the skin to turn red.

UV filters—another term for sunscreen chemicals that absorb UV rays.

vehicles (AKA carriers)—cosmetic compounds used to dilute an active ingredient, regulate its penetration into the skin, and/or help its surface application. It has been observed that the degree of ingredient effectiveness varies according to the vehicle used. This is called the "vehicle effect." In sunscreens, for example, the same amount of an active material in an oil or alcohol vehicle is less effective than the same material in a lotion vehicle, and this in turn is less effective than using a cream vehicle. The term *vehicle* also refers to components used in a cosmetic that provide the formulation with stability or consistency. A formulation can have one or more vehicles. Many times a vehicle may also be an active principle (e.g., alcohol).

vitamins—included in skin care products for a variety of performance and marketing reasons. Some vitamins, such as vitamin E, are considered to provide antioxidant properties. Though vitamins are considered natural materials by most consumers, in cosmetics they can be either naturally derived or synthetically produced. Some of the synthetic versions are more stable and easier to work with than their natural counterparts. There is a great deal of controversy over the difference of topical effectiveness between naturally derived versus synthetically formulated material. Thus far no definite conclusion has been reached.

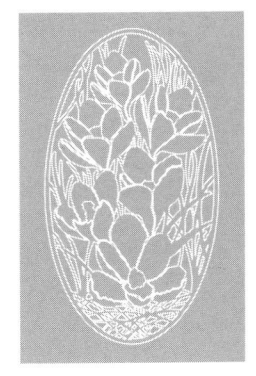

Part II
PRODUCT INGREDIENTS

INTRODUCTION

This dictionary represents the authors' analysis of cosmetic ingredients presently found on labels of skin care products. To compile this information the authors requested ingredient labels from U.S. manufacturers and importers of skin care products. These ingredients, plus others noted for use in skin care product formulation, were then alphabetically listed. Ingredient functions were analyzed based on published data, information provided by manufacturers, and interviews with cosmetic chemists from ingredient manufacturing companies. No data on product performance was directly obtained from cosmetic companies. This was specifically done to avoid the risk of describing product performance based on marketing claims.

Upon listing the cosmetic ingredients we discovered that there is no universal pattern used for listing product ingredients. In the case of botanicals, for example, some companies list them according to their Latin name, others by their English name (there may be more than one), and still others list them according to some traditional form of reference. The choice among the many possibilities depends on individual company preference.

To maintain uniformity, all botanicals have been listed and described in the dictionary by their primary English name, with most other names listed immediately after. Acacia, for example, can be found listed under A, as "**acacia** (AKA acacia gum; black catechu; gum acacia; gum arabic....)" To assist the reader with a botanical's Latin name, an alphabetical cross reference has been compiled in the appendix on page 321. For example, listed under A is "*Acacia senegal*—acacia." Another example is horse chestnut with a Latin name of *Aesculus hippocastanum*. It is listed and described in the main body of the dictionary under H for horse chestnut and found in the appendix under A for *Aesculus hippocastanum*.

When it comes to the chemical names of cosmetic ingredients, some companies list them according to their Cosmetic Toiletry and Fragrance Association (CTFA) name, considered the "official" name by cosmetic chemists. Others are listed by their chemical name and others by some form of abbreviation. When the name is a compound of more than one word, it could be listed by one company using those words in one order, by another in a reverse order, and by another either partially or fully abbreviated. Finally, some ingredients are listed under a trade name designated by the manufacturer to protect the proprietary nature of the formulation. Chemicals are also found listed by a marketing name that prevents the identification of its chemical composition.

An effort has been made in this dictionary to list chemical names under as many different forms as are found on product labels. The ingredient function, however, is discussed under its CTFA name or its most common form of reference. Other names for the same chemical are listed with a note to refer to the chemical's listed CTFA name for description. For example, butylated hydroxyanisole is commonly known and referred to as BHA. This ingredient is listed under both forms of reference but described only under BHA since this is the most common. Another example is benzophenone-3, also known as oxybenzone. It is listed and described under benzophenone-3 but can also be found under oxybenzone with a reference to the first ingredient for description.

Ingredients listed under a company trade name are referenced both ways and described under their chemical name whenever the chemical component was disclosed or could be determined.

An example is Ajidew. This is a trade name for sodium PCA, also listed as NaPCA (Na is the chemical symbol for sodium). In this case Ajidew is listed under A with a reference to sodium PCA for the description of ingredient properties.

In some instances certain ingredients perform very similar functions. Their inclusion in a formulation is determined by their reaction with other ingredients present, formulator's preference, and/or cost. In such cases a description is presented under one ingredient and all others are referenced to it. This is the case, with certain PEGs and laureths. For example, PEG 10 sorbitan laurate is a cleansing and solubilizing solution agent. PEG 40 sorbitan laurate, PEG 44 sorbitan laurate, PEG 75 sorbitan laurate, and PEG 80 sorbitan laurate are all referred to PEG 10 sorbitan laurate since they have a similar function.

Some ingredients are listed for marketing effect. Take for example fango mud. *Fango* is the term for mud in Italian; its description is found under mud. Other listings leave room for broad interpretation without real identification of the ingredient(s). Vague and marketing-oriented terms, whenever obvious, were noted in the dictionary. An example is active botanical fractions listed under A. This is a description involving two or more unidentified plant extracts, which precludes determining the ingredient's performance.

For some ingredients, minute quantities and low concentrations are an absolute requirement for appropriate skin response. For others, low concentrations render them ineffective. In addition, other ingredients present in a formulation may impact performance and bioavailability of certain active components. When it comes to the value of effectiveness as stated on labels or promotional material, in some cases the only way to be sure is based on the reputation and reliability of the cosmetic's manufacturer. Neither this book's authors nor an ingredient label reader is in a position to determine ingredient or product effectiveness based on the sequence of ingredients listed.

Ingredient manufacturers have stated time and time again that in many cases, especially with certain botanicals and new ingredients, some of the listing is more for marketing purposes than for a therapeutic effect since the concentration present may be too low for the ingredient's ascribed therapeutic attributes to actually be effective. It is therefore important to note the requirements surrounding cosmetic labeling. This will help with understanding the motivation and/or rationale behind labeling idiosyncracies.

COSMETIC INGREDIENT LABELING REGULATIONS

Today's cosmetic ingredient labeling regulations were established by the FDA in 1977. They require ingredients to be listed in descending order of predominance by the nomenclature established in reference sources of ingredient names. Flavor and fragrance ingredients need to be identified by the terms *flavor* and/or *fragrance,* as appropriate. Exempt from label disclosure under these regulations are the names of trade secret ingredients. A mechanism has been provided for the review of petitions for trade secret exemption. These regulations apply only to products for retail sale. Cosmetics used at professional establishments (e.g., salons or skin care clinics) or samples distributed free of charge cannot fall under the requirement of ingredient declaration.

Ingredient listings are printed on or affixed to product packaging. If a product is packaged in two containers, commonly bottle, tube, or jar housed in a box, it is required that the ingredients be printed on the package label of the outside container. Consider a cleanser sold in a box—the ingredient listing needs to appear on the box. Any listing on the bottle is optional. However, if an outer container is not used then the listing needs to appear on the main container, in this case, on the cleanser bottle. Such listings may appear on any information panel of a package displayed under customer conditions of purchase or on a tag, tape, or card firmly attached to a small size container. The regulation specifies that the information must be prominent, conspicuous, and clear.

Ingredients listed must be identified by the name established by the commissioner of the FDA for the purpose of ingredient labeling. If a name has not been established by the commissioner they must be identified by the name adopted for the ingredient in the editions and supplements of the following sources (listed in descending order of priority utilization):

- *CTFA Cosmetic Ingredient Dictionary*
- *United States Pharmacopoeia*
- *National Formulary*
- *Food Chemical Codex*
- *USAN and the USP Dictionary of Drug Names*

Theoretically, if an ingredient name is not listed in any of these sources, the name generally recognized by consumers or a chemical or technical name or description must be used. In reality, companies choose different means of labeling for the same ingredient, and many times names are slightly adapted for marketing purposes—fango mud is a prime example. Another example is the listing of bee pollen wax rather than the more common beeswax.

This becomes especially confusing when referring to herbal compounds. In some instances these compounds are listed by their botanical name and in others by their consumer or CTFA name. The issue can be further complicated by the way cosmetic manufacturing companies choose to spell the ingredients used. They may elect to spell out the name, as in the case of pyrodixine hydrochloride, and dihydroxyacetone, or use chemical symbols or acronyms as part of or as a replacement for the whole name. Hence, pyrodixine hydrochloride might be found listed as pyrodixine HCl and dihydroxyacetone as DHA. To facilitate label interpretation this dictionary cross references as many such instances as feasible.

That ingredients in a formulation be listed in descending order of predominance is to comply with the Fair Packaging and Labeling (FP&L) Act. One exception is that if a cosmetic is also a drug the active drug ingredient(s) must be listed before the cosmetic ones. Each drug ingredient must be declared as an "active ingredient" and identified by its established drug name.

The second exception to the order of predominance rule is that if an ingredient is accorded confidentiality as a trade secret by the FDA, a listing of "other ingredients" may be used at the end of the declaration instead of the ingredient's actual name(s). Rather than list "other ingredients," some companies list an ingredient or group of ingredients considered proprietary under an assumed company name, which does not allow its identification through any of the listed sources. Companies must submit an application to the FDA for their ingredient(s) to have trade secret status. The Freedom of Information Act states, "A trade secret may consist of any formula, pattern, device or compilation of information which is used in one's business and which gives him an opportunity to obtain an advantage over competitors who do not know or use it." In other words, a trade secret is information of value not known to others and that cannot be readily ascertained.

The labeling regulation permits ingredients present at 1% concentrations or lower to be listed in any order, as long as they appear after the ingredients present at higher concentrations in their order of predominance. Color additives present at any concentration may be listed in any order after the listing of ingredients that are not color additives.

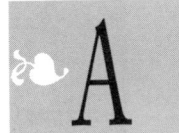

acacia *(Acacia senegal)* (AKA acacia gum; black catechu; gum acacia; gum Arabic)—commonly used in old-time remedies as a soothing and anti-inflammatory agent. In extract form, acacia is recommended for dry, sensitive, or delicate skin. It is also used as a vegetable gum for product thickening. Acacia is the dried, gummy sap from the stems and branches of various species of the African acacia tree. It may cause skin rashes due to allergy.

acacia gum—*see* acacia.

acerola—a rich source of ascorbic acid. It can function as an antioxidant and anti-free radical. Acerola is derived from the ripe fruit of the West Indies or Barbados cherry variety.

acetamide MEA (AKA ethanol acetamide)—a humectant recommended for use in emulsions. According to manufacturers it has counterirritant properties.

acetate—a salt of acetic acid. Although found listed on labels as acetate, to determine its appropriate action it needs to be followed or preceded by another name (e.g. acetate tocopherol). The second name determines the compound's function.

acetone—a solvent considered to be a noncomedogenic (not producing comedones) ingredient occasionally used in skin toners. It could be drying and very irritating to the skin depending on the concentration and frequency of use.

acetylated lanolin—an emollient that helps form water-repellent films on the skin.

acetylated lanolin alcohol—exhibits skin-softening and anti-allergenic properties. This is an ester resembling steroids generally found on the skin. Considered highly comedogenic (producing comedones or blackheads) by some sources, with only a mild irritancy potential.

Achillea **extract**—*see* yarrow extract.

acrylamide copolymer—has a film-forming capability and is similar to acrylates copolymer. Acrylamide copolymer is a polymer of two or more monomers consisting of an acrylamide and/or its simple alkyl derivative.

acrylates—*see* acrylates copolymer.

acrylates copolymer—is able to absorb skin secretions, thereby reducing skin shine and providing an improved skin surface for makeup applications. Acrylates copolymer also imparts a pleasant feel to the cosmetic preparation and helps reduce any feeling of oiliness the product may have. Its various applications include incorporation into skin cleansers, oil control treatments, makeups, and loose and compressed powders. Used with a variety of other ingredients, including glycerin, cyclomethicone, retinyl palmitate, and vegetable oils, acrylates copolymer prolongs the availability to the skin of these other ingredients through a time-release type of activity. It also helps either counteract some negative properties they may have when applied to the skin or further enhance their positive ones. For example, acrylates copolymer reduces the tackiness and greasiness of glycerin while prolonging its availability in the interstitial network of the skin. When present with retinyl palmitate, acrylates copolymer improves the stability of vitamin A palmitate formulations and increases its skin contact time.

acrylates/C$_{10-30}$ alkyl acrylate copolymer—an emulsifier for oil-in-water emulsions with thickening and formula-stabilizing properties similar to a carbomer. It allows for release of the formulation's oil phase component immediately upon rubbing the product into the skin. Used in moisturizer emulsions and creams, waterproof sunscreens, and fragrance emulsions.

acrylates/C$_{10-30}$ alkyl acrylate crosspolymer—*see* acrylates/C$_{10-30}$ alkyl acrylate copolymer.

acrylates/t-octylpropenamide copolymer—has moisture barrier as well as waterproofing/water-repelling properties. It is commonly found in skin care products requiring a film-forming component, including waterproof sunscreens, smudge-proof eye products, and hand and body moisturizers. Studies indicate that this ingredient allows for the gradual release of active principles over a period of time. Other properties include rub-off resistance and fragrance retention.

acrylic acid/acrylonitogens copolymer—used as a primary emulsifier. It modifies the feel of gels and emulsions to give the sensation of a natural product. It is found in preparations requiring waterproofing properties.

acrylic acid polymers—can be employed as thickeners, dispersion stabilizers, and viscosity modifiers for cosmetics. Clinical studies indicate no dermal reactions or irritations.

active botanical fractions—this ingredient listing is accompanied by a claim that the mixture combines anti-elastase of active plant fractions and therefore can be used for preserving elastin. However, this is a vague listing involving two or more unidentified botanical extracts, which precludes determining the ingredient's appropriate or actual value.

adenosine phosphate—a nucleotide (building blocks of nucelic acid) added to skin care products to bind water and moisture.

agrimony extract *(Agrimonia eupatoria)*—astringent. Considered a beneficial botanical ingredient for use in toners.

AHA—*see* alpha hydroxyacid.

Ajidew—*see* sodium PCA.

Ajidew A-100—*see* PCA.

Ajidew N-50—*see* sodium PCS.

alanine—an amino acid that can act as a skin-conditioning agent. Usually used in combination with other amino acids.

alchemilla extract *(Alchemilla vulgaris)* (AKA lady's mantle)—according to contemporary phytotherapy, alchemilla is beneficial for wound healing and inflammation. It is also credited with anti-free radical and UV filtering properties. *See also* lady's mantle extract.

alcohol (AKA alcohol SD-40; alcohol SDA-40; ethanol; ethyl alcohol)—widely used in the cosmetic industry as an antiseptic as well as a solvent given its strong grease-dissolving abilities. Often used in a variety of concentrations in skin toners for acne skin, aftershave lotions, perfumes, suntan lotions, and toilet waters. Alcohol is drying to the skin when used in high concentrations. It is manufactured via the fermentation of starch, sugar, and other carbohydrates.

alcohols benzoate/C-12-15—an emulsifier with application in sun-protection lotions. This is a mixture of synthetic aliphatic alcohols.

alcohol SD-40 (AKA SD alcohol 40)—"SD" is the acronym for "specially denatured." This is a high-grade version of ethyl alcohol designed especially for cosmetic use. It evaporates almost immediately, leaving the active ingredients on the surface. Antibactericidal properties are ascribed to it. The number 40 does not relate to the percentage of alcohol in the formulation but to the alcohol's grade. *See also* alcohol.

alcohol SDA-40—another way of describing alcohol SD-40. This could be read as "alcohol, special denatured alcohol." *See also* alcohol SD-40.

aleppo gall (AKA oak bud extract)—an active botanical substance used in sun products due to its anti-free radical, UV filter, and skin repair activities in cases of UV ray damage. Aleppo gall helps combat the harmful effects of UVA rays and protects the skin given its UVB filtering abilities. It also has astringent and antiseptic properties, making it useful for treating burns and healing wounds. Traditionally, allepo gall was also used in the treatment of eczema.

alfalfa extract *(Medicago sativa)*—a botanical considered to have tonic and decongestant properties. Alfalfa is a widely cultivated perennial plant that can also be found growing wild on the borders of fields and in low valleys. The extract is obtained from the leaves.

algae extract (AKA seaweed extract)—an active substance used to normalize the skin's moisture content and provide suppleness to the epidermis. There are many varieties of algae, and they exhibit different properties including anti-free radical properties. Manufacturers rarely disclose the specific strain of algae being employed. This often remains as part of the formulation's "secret." *See also* seaweed extract.

algae oil—*see* algae extract; seaweed extract.

algae protein—studies are noting that some specific varieties are good substitutes for animal-derived collagen. They are also finding that algae protein has potentially better moisturizing benefits at lower levels of use and a reduced feeling of tackiness often associated with the higher use levels of animal-derived collagen. *See also* algae extract; seaweed extract.

algin—(AKA alginic acid; potassium alginate; sodium alginate)—used in cosmetic formulations as a thickener, stabilizer, and gelling agent. Obtained from different varieties of brown seaweed.

alginate—used as a thickening agent in cosmetic preparations. Alginate may be used as microcapsules and is obtained from marine extracts.

alginic acid—*see* algin.

allantoin—a botanical extract said to be healing and soothing. It is considered an excellent temporary antiirritant and is believed to aid in the healing of damaged skin by stimulating new tissue growth. Allantoin is appropriate for sensitive, irritated, and acne skins. Found in the comfrey root, it is considered nonallergenic.

almond flour—used primarily in soaps to give them a thicker consistency and scrub capability.

almond meal—used in cosmetic scrubs to achieve exfoliation. It does not have any other direct effect on the skin. It comes in different sieve sizes, #1 being very fine and #10 very large. Almond meal is made from the almond shell.

almond oil, bitter—serves as an emollient and a carrier, providing an elegant skin feel and promoting spreadability in creams, lotions, and bath oils. Obtained from the bitter almond, it supposedly stays fresh longer than oil obtained from sweet almonds. It is the volatile essential oil distilled from almonds and is also used in fragrance and flavors. When used in large quantities it is known to cause strong allergic reactions including headaches.

almond oil, sweet—serves as an emollient and a carrier, providing an elegant skin feel and promoting spreadability in creams, lotions, and bath oils. Sweet almond oil's main constituent is olein with a small proportion of glyceride of linoleic acid. It is very similar in composition to olive oil. It is obtained from sweet almonds that have undergone a cleaning and crushing process, which leaves them in powder form. The powder is then cold-pressed and left to "rest" for 1–2 weeks. After the resting period the almond oil is filtered and often bleached. Sweet almond oil is the triglyceride oil (vegetable oil) derived from almonds.

almond powder—*see* almond flour.

almond protein—has moisture-binding properties. Derived from almond meal.

almondermin—leaves skin with a velvety feel. It has moisturizing, smoothing, and soothing properties. Almondermin is a botanical extract mixture of sweet almonds and marshmallow.

aloe extract—a popular botanical recognized for centuries as having beneficial medicinal properties including antibiotic, anti-inflammatory, and wound healing. These benefits have been found to apply to skin care as well. Aloe vera is frequently used in cosmetic preparations due to its apparent moisturizing, soothing, and calming properties. It is excellent for dry and sensitive skin, as well as for the treatment of sunburns and other minor burns, insect bites, and skin irritations. Aloe extract is obtained from aloe vera leaves and is also referred to as aloe vera gel. *See also* aloe vera.

aloe juice—also referred to as aloe vera gel. Technically, the term *aloe juice* applies to a diluted version of aloe vera gel. *See also* aloe vera.

aloe vera *(Aloe vera)*—an emollient and film-forming gum resin with hydrating, softening, healing, antimicrobial, and anti-inflammatory properties. Its moisturizing ability is its most widely recognized characteristic. Aloe vera penetrates the skin, supplying moisture directly to the tissue. Other properties include moisture regulation and an apparent ability to absorb UV light. It has a slightly relaxing effect on the skin, making it beneficial for sensitive, sunburned, and sun-exposed skins. Aloe vera was popular in folklore medicine as a remedy for burns. It is frequently used in gels as an effective refresher and relaxer for irritated skin, hence its popularity in sun preparations for cooling and soothing. In addition, it is found to be an effective component in emulsions formulated for regulating dry skin. Apparently, aloe vera also has a synergistic effect when used in conjunction with other anti-inflammatory substances. Concentrations over 50% have been shown to increase the blood supply to the area of application. Though aloe vera's important constituents are minerals, polysaccharides, amino acids, and carbohydrates, it is constituted of about 99.5% water. Its benefit in a skin care product depends on a proper concentration, as different concentrations result in different benefits and end products. This almost odorless and nearly colorless extract is derived from the sap of the aloe leaf. It is used in the form of a gel (also referred to as an extract) or in a diluted version referred to as aloe vera juice.

aloe vera gel—the mucilage obtained from aloe vera leaves. *See also* aloe vera.

alpha hydroxyacid (AKA AHA)—an active substance with exfoliating and emollient properties. Under certain conditions AHA is also found to be moisturizing and hydrating. Its topical application seems to have specific, distinct, and unique effects on the corneum layer, the epidermis, the dermis, and the pilosebaceous follicle. The exfoliating and hyperkeratinization-reducing properties of some AHAs makes them prime ingredients for acne-oriented products, for reducing actinic keratosis, and for improving the appearance of aging skin. Also, AHA's emollient and skin hydration properties helps dry, irritated, and aged skin. Continuous use of some AHAs has helped in the smoothing of very fine wrinkles. Alpha hydroxyacid is the family name for a variety of acids including citric acid from citrus fruits, glycolic acid from sugar cane, lactic acid from sour milk, malic acid from apples, and tartaric acid from old wine. Until recently, when glycolic acid became the AHA of choice, the most common AHAs used in skin care preparations were lactic and citric acids.

Some Examples of AHAs				
Glycolic Acid	**Lactic Acid**	**Malic Acid**	**Tartaric Acid**	**Citric Acid**
CH_2OH	CH_3	$COOH$	$COOH$	$COOH$
$COOH$	$CHOH$	CH_2	$CHOH$	CH_2
	$COOH$	$CHOH$	$CHOH$	$HOC-COOH$
		$COOH$	$COOH$	CH_2
				$COOH$

Some examples of AHAs

alpha hydroxyacetic acid—*see* glycolic acid.

alpha hydroxycaproic acid—when added to sunscreen preparations it can prevent the skin peeling that results from excessive sun exposure.

alpha hydroxyethanoic acid—*see* glycolic acid.

alpha tocopherol—*see* vitamin E.

althea extract *(Althaea officinalis)* (AKA marshmallow extract; marshmallow root extract)—botanical that is said to have emollient and soothing capabilities when incorporated into skin care formulations. It is considered beneficial in aftershave preparations and in products for treating sunburns and dry skin. This is a natural hydroglycolic plant extract from the althea root.

alum—*see* potassium alum.

aluminum PCA—has astringent and antiseptic properties.

aluminum acetate solution (AKA Burow's solution)—has astringent and antiseptic properties and is used in astringent lotions and protective creams. This is a mixture of alkali metal acetate, acetic acid, and dibasic aluminium acetate with boric acid as a formula stabilizer. Some cosmetic companies try to avoid using this ingredient because of its metal content since the benefits of metal-based products on the skin are questioned by some manufacturers. Prolonged and continuous use can produce a skin rash and severe sloughing of the skin.

aluminum hydroxide gel—an inorganic compound serving as an opaquifying agent used in the formulation of facial masks and makeup preparations.

aluminum magnesium hydroxystearate—an additive and formula stabilizer generally applicable to water-in-oil emulsions. It helps improve the suspension of insoluble particles or pigments in formulations and is particularly useful when manufacturers desire a colorless gel.

aluminum starch octenyl succinate—an SPF enhancer, particularly when used in combination with titanium dioxide. It is hydrophobic (lacking affinity for water) and can be used to reduce the feeling of greasiness in a product.

aluminum stearate—a saline form of stearic acid used as a thickener and emulsifier and to regulate the stability and suspension of a cosmetic formulation. This aluminum stearic acid soap can be found in coconut and vegetable oils.

aluminum sulfate—a common aluminum salt used in astringents. It is very similar to aluminum.

amino acid—used in cosmetic formulations to enhance water retention and skin moisturization. Because of their reduced size, amino acids can penetrate deeper into the stratum corneum's cell layers than proteins with a higher molecular weight, such as collagen. The ingredient's "feel" on the skin will depend on the amino acid composition of the protein used. Though the most commonly used amino acids are derived from animal collagen, due to consumer demand new vegetable substitutes are being introduced, and ongoing investigations are seeking alternative sources. Although amino acids are fundamental skin components, the skin does not utilize topically applied amino acids to produce new skin as the formation of skin from amino acids is an extremely complex process.

ρ-aminobenzoic acid (AKA PABA)—a sunscreen chemical with an approved usage level of 5–15%. It is found irritating to sensitive skin, has the potential to cause sensitization, and is considered too water soluble. Once extremely popular, this ingredient has all but disappeared from sunscreen formulations. PABA is a yellowish or colorless acid found in vitamin B complex.

aminoethyl propanol—an alcohol with antibactericidal and topical antiseptic properties generally used as a pH adjuster in cosmetic formulations.

aminomethyl propanol—an alcohol used as a pH adjuster in cosmetic formulations. Its primary application is in hair preparations.

aminoserine—*see* serine.

ammonium alpha hydroxyethanoate — *see* ammonium glycolate.

ammonium chloride—used as a thickener and as an additive in nonalcoholic toners. According to cosmetic formulators, the ammonium component provides the tingling or stinging sensation that some people associate with toners or aftershaves, and which, in regular toners, is usually provided by the alcohol content. Ammonium chloride's use is the result of preference in formulation feel.

ammonium cocoyl isethionate—a surfactant. Its mildness and high-foaming property give a product a lubricative lather and a soft skin feel. It is derived from natural coconut oil.

ammonium glycolate—basically a cleanser used in shampoos and liquid soaps. Ammonium glycolate is also a neutralized version of glycolic acid commonly incorporated in glycolic-acid-based cosmetics to reduce the irritation typically associated with the use of free glycolic acid. *See also* glycolic acid.

ammonium hydroxide—used in cosmetic preparations as an alkali to neutralize excessive acidity in a formulation.

ammonium lactate—when topically applied it is found to thicken the epidermis while reducing the thickness of the corneum layer. A neutralized version of lactic acid. *See also* lactic acid.

ammonium lauryl sulfate—a surfactant with emulsifying capabilities. Given its detergent properties, it can be used, at mild acidic pH levels, as an anionic surfactant cleanser. It can cause skin irritation.

amniotic fluid—some consider this simply an animal protein serving as a surface film-forming agent with moisturizing properties. Others claim it is nourishing to the skin, has antitoxic properties, acts as an epithelial stimulant, and has a transcutaneous diffusion factor. Controversies over such claims are extended to frozen versus unfrozen versions of the ingredient. Research indicates that amniotic fluid, like other animal extracts, seems to have a positive effect on wound healing and cellular regeneration. Advocates of its use versus other animal extracts further point out that animal sacrifice is not required to obtain the substance, since the amniotic fluid (the fluid surrounding the cow embryo in utero) can be extracted from live animals in their third to sixth month of gestation supposedly without harm to the animal or fetus.

amodimethicone copolyol—a silicone product with skin softening and conditioning properties.

amphoteric 2—an extremely mild surfactant commonly used in baby shampoos. It can also serve as an excellent emulsifier.

amydimethyl PABA—a chemical UVB absorbed. It is no longer available in the United States as production has ceased due to reports of skin sensitivity.

anemone extract (*Anemone* sp.)—a botanical ingredient with soothing and anti-inflammatory properties as well as the ability to heal superficial wounds. These attributes would make it appropriate for sensitive, delicate, and acne skin. There are about 70 species of anemone. Most frequently used are wood anemone *(Anemone nemorosa)* and the pasque flower *(Anemone pulstilla)*. Some varieties of anemone are known to cause swelling and blistering. The extract is obtained from the whole herb.

angelica *(Angelica* sp.)—in both extract and essential oil form, this botanical is described as tonic, detoxifying, and purifying for the blood and lymph systems. Angelica's principal constituents are volatile oil (about 1%), valeric acid, angelic acid, sugar, a bitter principle, and a peculiar resin called angelicin that is stimulating to the skin. The essential oil of the root contains terebangelene and other terpenes. The oils of the seeds contain methyl-ethylacetic acid and hydroxymyristic acid. Angelica extracts are made from the seeds and, more often, the roots.

anhydrous lanolin—an emollient and emulsifying agent that, depending on its processing, may be a comedogenic or noncomedogenic ingredient. *See also* lanolin.

animal collagen amino acids—amino acids derived from animal collagen. *See also* amino acid; collagen; protein.

animal protein derivative—*see* protein.

animal red blood cells extract—considered a metabolic activator. Studies indicate this extract has the ability to stimulate oxygen absorption. It is used in cosmetic creams and aftershave products due to an ability to accelerate minor cut and burn healing, and because it seems to increase blood circulation in the skin. It usually comprises about 1% of cosmetic formulation, although to measure oxygen absorption activity the concentration must be about 3%.

animal tissue extract—an animal protein extracted from the dermis, testes, and ovaries of the pig and the thymus, placenta, and mammae of the cow. *See also* protein.

anise extract *(Pimpinella anisum)*—used as a fragrance. No therapeutic value has been ascribed to the external application of this botanical. Anise's composition is 80–90% anethole and methyl claricol. The extract is obtained by steam distillation of the anise seeds. It may cause allergic reactions and produce hives, scaling, and blisters when applied directly to the skin.

annatto extract *(Bixa orellana)*—used in creams and sun products as a colorant and a highlighter. It is an orange color obtained from the plant's dried fruit, specifically the pulp.

apple extract *(Pyrus malus)*—claimed by some to have soothing properties and be beneficial for dry skin. Fresh apples and apple juice contain malic and tartaric acid, which can exfoliate the skin to some degree, and the enzyme aneylase. Aneylase's properties in cosmetic preparations are unknown. As vitamin and enzymatic actions are easily destroyed, the value of the vitamin content and enzymatic action of the fruit in cosmetic preparations is totally dependent on the product's formulation.

apricot oil—*see* apricot kernel oil.

apricot kernel oil—an emollient with a nongreasy feel. It provides good slip and lubricity to a product. Primarily used as a carrier, apricot kernel oil is a good moisturizing and occlusive agent and finds considerable use in cosmetics for its skin-softening action. This oil is rapidly absorbed by the skin and has a high vitamin E content (*see* vitamin E), that some claim can aid the skin in retaining elasticity, clarity, and suppleness. Apricot kernel oil is a triglyceride in the same category as avocado oil, olive oil, and sesame oil and is comprised of approximately 75% oleic acid and 20% linoleic acid—unsaturated fatty acids esterified with glycerin. Apricot kernel oil is considered by some chemists to be a natural replacement for mineral oil. It is extracted from the apricot kernel by expression and is far less expensive than almond oil, which it very closely resembles and can therefore substitute.

apricot powder—a natural peeling material incorporated into soaps and scrubs.

apricot seeds—the seeds are ground and then incorporated into soaps and scrubs as a natural peeling material.

apricot stone (ground)—*see* apricot powder.

arachidonic acid—an ingredient with skin-smoothing, emollient, and healing properties. Arachidonic acid is an essential fatty acid present in the skin and considered critical for appropriate skin metabolism. Most that is used for cosmetic purposes is animal derived.

arachidyl propionate—aids in the rapid spreadability of a cosmetic preparation. It has a nonoily feel and a high sheen. A noncomedogenic, semisolid ester that liquifies at body temperature. Some consider it a possible replacement for lanolin.

arachis oil (AKA peanut oil)—a carrier oil used in cosmetic products designed for sensitive and delicate skin. *See also* peanut oil.

l-arginine—an amino acid used as a skin conditioning agent. *See also* amino acid.

arginine PCA—in a cosmetic preparation it appears to have the ability to increase the skin's oxygen consumption and improve moisturization.

Arlacel (165)—very good, acid-stable emulsifier. It keeps the oil and water molecules together to maintain a product's integrity and has no effect on the skin. Arlacel is a trade name for a glyceryl stearate and PEG 100 stearate mixture.

armoise oil—a mixture of natural essential oils said to have antimicrobial properties and the ability to act as a cosmetic preservative. For this mixture to be effective in a cosmetic preparation, a 2% concentration is required. Mixtures such as these in leave-on products may cause skin sensitivity if not carefully formulated.

arnica extract *(Arnica montana)*—a botanical credited with a wide variety of properties including antiseptic, astringent, antimicrobial, anti-inflammatory, anticoagulant, circulation stimulating, healing, and stimulating. Some claim it promotes the removal of wastes from the skin, aids in the promotion of new tissue growth, and is anti-allergenic. Traditionally used upon appearance of couperose condition, arnica extract is also considered excellent for an acne condition. It is effective in gels and creams designed to treat damaged, reddened, or tired skin. Important constituents include arnicin, a volatile oil, tannin, phulin, sesquiterpenes, flavonoids, and courmarins. The flowers of this perennial herb are said to contain more arnicin than the rhizome and are the preferred segment of the plant used. Repeated applications may produce severe inflammation, and great care must be exercised in its use as some people are particularly sensitive to the plant.

arnica oil—credited with healing properties. *See also* arnica extract.

artichoke extract *(Cynara scolymus)*—sources claim that artichoke extract helps heal skin irritations and is anti-inflammatory and beautifying. Studies also indicate that artichoke extract leaves dry skin more vital, smoother, and firmer with an improvement at the dermal level. In cases of oily skin it seems to help regulate oiliness, clear the skin, and cause pores to appear smaller. According to studies, it can also help even out skin tone and improve blemished complexions. Important constituents include tannin, pectin, and glucoside compounds.

ascophyllum algae—a type of algea. *See* algae extract.

ascorbic acid (AKA vitamin C)—Ascorbic acid and its derivatives, such as ascorbyl linoleate, are said to have skin-lightening and antioxidant properties. Its stability is a main concern among formulators when incorporating it into cosmetic formulations. *See also* vitamin C.

l-ascorbic acid ethylene oxide—an adduct with skin-lightening properties. Tests indicate that it inhibits melanin formation.

ascorbyl linoleate—an ascorbic acid derivative. It serves as a skin-lightening agent or inhibits skin darkening by preventing melanin formation.

ascorbyl palmitate—used as a preservative and an antioxidant in cosmetic creams and lotions to prevent rancidity. Ascorbyl palmitate facilitates the incorporation of ingredients such as vitamins A, D, and C into cosmetic formulations. It has no known toxicity.

ascorbyl polypeptide—an ingredient that allows for better incorporation of vitamin C into cosmetic preparations.

asebiol—said to regulate excessive oil gland activity, aid in emulsifying excess sebum, possess skin-softening properties, and promote surface skin peeling. This is a mixture based on hydrolized yeast extract containing lipopeptides and phospholipids to which sulfuric amino acids, water-soluble vitamin B, urea, methionin, and cysterin have been added.

l-aspartic acid—an amino acid used as a skin-conditioning agent. *See also* aspartic acid.

aspartic acid—an amino acid used to give skin smoothness. It is usually present in products for dry skin. Aspartic acid is a nonessential amino acid naturally occurring in animals, plants, sugar cane, sugar beets, and molasses. A synthetic version is more commonly used for commercial applications.

Australian tea tree oil *(Melaleuca alternifolia)*—*see* tea tree oil.

avens extract *(Geum urbanum)*—A botanical credited with antiseptic and skin-clearing properties. For therapeutic properties the extract is obtained from the roots of the herb.

avocado oil—can function as an emollient and as a carrier oil in a cosmetic preparation, helping transport active substances into the skin. Its skin-benefiting properties include bactericidal and soothing, particularly to sensitive skin. Current speculation among researchers is that avocado oil may mobilize and increase the collagen of connective tissue. This would keep the skin moist and smooth in addition to having a favorable influence in the treatment for minor skin conditions. Avocado oil has also demonstrated sunscreening characteristics and has been given the highest ranking by the *Encyclopedia of Chemical Technology* for sunscreen effectiveness when compared to other naturally derived oils such as peanut, olive, and coconut. In cosmetic formulations it is also employed to help stabilize oil-in-water emulsions and can be effectively used in cleansing creams, moisturizers, lipsticks, makeup bases, bath oils, sunscreen, and suntan preparations. Avocado oil enjoys the highest penetration rate among similar oils (corn, soybean, olive, and almond). It consists mostly of oleic, linoleic, and linolenic acids. Other constituents include palmitic and palmitoleic acids, lecithin, phytosterol, carotinoids, and a high concentration of vitamins A, D, and E. This oil is obtained from the ripe avocado fruit and is generally expressed from the seed.

avocado oil (unsaponifiable)—has excellent penetration and sunscreening properties. *See also* avocado oil.

azulene—renowned as an anti-inflammatory and soothing agent. Excellent for sensitive skin, azulene is a German chamomile derivative with a characteristic deep blue color. Careful—it stains! *See also* chamomile.

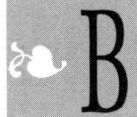

babassu oil—a superior emollient. Babassu oil is exceptional for use in sunscreen products, and beneficial for combination skin as it offers mildness to the dry skin areas without furthering the oiliness of an already oily T-zone.

baking soda—*see* sodium bicarbonate.

balm—*see* balm mint extract.

balm of Gilead *(Commiphora meccanensis, Commiphora opobalsamum)*—helps in treatment of eczema and dry skin.

balm mint extract *(Melissa officinalis)* (AKA balm; melissa)—folklore ascribes the following properties to balm: "revivifying a man completely, effective for treating nervous disorders, strengthen the brain, relieves languishing nature."[1] Modern research, on the other hand, is a bit more specific, attributing calming, soothing, healing, antispasmodic, tightening, antibactericidal, and circulation stimulating properties to balm mint. It can be beneficially incorporated into acne treatment formulations and postsun preparations, with positive action in products for blemished or sensitive skins as well. Balm mint's effectiveness is due to its constituents that include citral, citronella, linalol, geraliol and aldehydes. Its strong aroma makes it a popular fragrance component. Derived from the leaf or leaf juice.

---

1. Mrs. M. Grieve, *A Modern Herbal* (New York: Dover Publications, Inc., 1971)

balm mint oil (AKA, balsam; lemon balm; melissa oil)—the general effects attributed to this oil include sedative, antispasmodic, and antiseptic. Its use is indicated for acne skin and for individuals with dermatitis and eczema conditions. Laboratory studies have established the presence of caffeic acid, rosemary acid, salicylic acid, luteolin, and apigenin. Sugar constituents such as glucose and maltose have also been identified, along with amino acids such as proline, asparogine, glutonine acid, valien, serine, alanine, and methionine. The recommended use level for this oil is 1–10% of a formulation's total composition. Balm mint oil has a very low yield and, as a result, is a very expensive oil. Because of this it is widely adulterated, usually with citronella and lemongrass. The oil is obtained from the leaves and tops of *Melissa officinalis*. There are some indications that balm mint oil may cause skin irritation.

balsam—*see* balm mint oil.

balsam Peru *(Myroxylon pereirae)*—a botanical to which strong medicinal actions are attributed. It is recommended for cases of scabies and skin diseases. It is also considered antibacterial and is preferred by some to sulfur ointments. In addition, it has been considered of value in later stages of acute eczema. Balsam Peru is recommended for use on acne skin conditions and eczema. Its main constituents are a colorless, aromatic, oily liquid called cinnamein; a dark resin known as peruviol; a small quantity of vanillin; and cinnamic acid. It is extracted from the trunk of a large and beautiful tree, akin to mahogany. Every part of the tree, including the leaves, abounds in a resinous juice.

balsam tolu oil *(Myrospermum toluiferum)*—valuable to perfumers as a fixative. Its botanical actions are mostly indicated for internal use and its value in external applications is not clear. It is described as a stimulant. This oil is constituted of about 80% amorphous resin, with cinnamic acid and a little vanillin, benzyl benzoate, and benzyl cinnamate. It is sometimes used instead of balsam Peru. It is obtained by making V-shaped cuts in the tree.

bamboo extract—used in cosmetics for its moisture-binding properties.

banana oil (AKA plantain fruit)—a carrier oil. The banana family is of more interest for its nutrient than for its botanical properties. The use of plantain juice as an antidote for snake bites has been reported in parts of Southeast Asia since 1916.

barberry extract *(Berberis vulgaris)*—its herbal properties have been reported as anti-inflammatory, antiseptic, and beneficial for application to cutaneous eruptions. The common barberry is a bushy shrub cultivated for its fruit, but the stembark and rootbark are used for cosmetic applications. Barberry bark's main constituent is berberine, a bitter alkaloid. Other constituents include oxyacanthine, berbamine, other alkaloidal matter, a little tannin, wax, resin, fat, albumin, gum, and starch.

bardane extract (AKA burdock)—*see* burdock root extract.

barium sulfate—an inorganic salt with very little use in cosmetics. It is more commonly used for making noncosmetic soaps.

barley oil *(Hordeum vulgare)*—a carrier oil with soothing properties.

basil oil *(Ocimum basilicum)*—physicians of old were unable to agree on its medicinal value, some declaring that it was a poison and others describing it as a precious simple. Its herbal action is described as aromatic and carminative. Although the value of its topical application other than as a carrier oil is not clear, it could be described as stimulating, tonic, and purifying.

batyl alcohol—an emulsion stabilizer and occlusive skin-conditioning agent. The mono-octadecyl ether of glycerin.

bayberry *(Myrica cerifera)*—its properties are described as astringent, antibacterial, and stimulant. Bayberry's application is primarily for acne and damaged skin. The parts of the plant used are the dried bark of the root and the wax. Volatile oil, starch, lignin, gum, albumen, extractive, tannic and gallic acids, acrid and astringent resins, a red coloring substance, and an acid resembling saponin are all constituents that have been found in the stem bark and the root. The wax consists of the glycerides of stearic, palmitic, and myristic acids and a small quantity of oleaic acid. Bayberry is another name for the wild cinnamon found in the West Indies and South America that yields oil of bayberry.

bean oil *(Phaseolus vulgaris)*—a carrier. Found to be soothing and relieve itching. Bean oil is said to be good for skins with an acne condition.

bearberry extract *(Arctostaphylus uva-urusi)*—the leaves have a powerful astringency and probably also an antiseptic and anti-inflammatory effect. The main constituent of bearberry leaves is a crystallizable glucoside called arbutin. Other constituents include methy-arbutin, ericolin, ursone, gallic acid, ellagic acid, and probably also myriceting. The bearberry plant is a small shrub, and the dried leaves are the only part of the plant used in cosmetics.

beech tree extract *(Fagus sylvatica)*—it is claimed by herbologists that, when used in proper form, beech tree extract increases protein synthesis and enzymatic activity of keratinocytes. Other properties, such as stimulating and antiseptic, are also attributed to the beech tar making it of value for application in various skin diseases. The oil is used in the same fashion as other fixed oils and is considered a carrier. Well-ripened beech nuts, called "mast," yield 17–20% of a nondrying oil similar to hazel and cottonseed oils.

beer yeast (natural)—*see* yeast.

bee pollen wax—*see* beeswax.

beeswax—one of the oldest raw ingredients used in cosmetic preparations. Its applications are many. It has traditionally been used as an emulsifier for water-in-oil emulsions and is now also used to regulate a formulation's consistency. Beeswax is used as part of the wax composition of solid and paste products such as creams, lipsticks, and pomades. When on the skin's surface it can form a network rather than a film as is the case with petrolatum. Though there is no scientific proof for it, beeswax is credited with anti-inflammatory, antiallergic, antioxidant, antibactericidal, germicidal, and skin-softening and elasticity-enhancing properties. As an antioxidant beeswax has some free-radical-scavenging ability. Depending on its source, beeswax can be considered a noncomedogenic ingredient. It rarely causes sensitivity, and allergic reactions to beeswax are low.

beeswax (white)—regular beeswax that has been bleached. Unbleached beeswax is yellow. *See also* beeswax.

beeswax (liquid paraffin)—*see* beeswax.

beet powder *(Beta vulgaris)*—used mostly for color.

behenic acid—this is a long-chain fatty acid used in product formulations to form a viscous emulsion. Considered a noncomedogenic raw material.

behenoxy dimethicone—an emollient, pigment dispersant, lubricant, and moisture barrier silicone. It is used in small quantities to give smooth slip on the skin.

behenyl alcohol—a binder and an emulsion stabilizer. Used also to increase a formulation's viscosity. This is a mixture of fatty alcohols.

behenyl erucate—an occlusive skin-conditioning agent. Considered noncomedogenic.

behenyl triglyceride—a skin-conditioning agent. Considered a noncomedogenic raw material.

bentonite (AKA bentonite clay)—used to regulate the viscosity and suspension properties of a cosmetic formulation. It also acts as an overall formula stabilizer. Bentonite's water absorption capabilities allow it to form a gelatinous mass. It is used in face masks because of its properties as a suspending agent. Bentonite, considered a noncomedogenic raw material, is a colloidal aluminum silicate clay.

bentonite clay—*see* bentonite.

benzalkonium chloride—a preservative. With continuous use it can cause occasional allergic reactions.

benzethonium chloride—a preservative that works against algae, bacteria, and fungi. In skin care preparations it is safe for use at concentrations of 0.5%.

benzoic acid—a preservative primarily for use against molds and yeasts. Its performance is classified only as fair against bacteria. Benzoic acid is used in concentrations of 0.05–0.1%. Although it has a low sensitizing rate, it may cause an allergic reaction in persons sensitive to similar chemicals.

benzoin—a fragrant essential oil with bactericidal, anti-irritation, and anti-itching properties. It is considered a good ingredient for reducing skin redness and is also a preservative of fats. While its primary constituent is benzoic acid, it also contains canillin and an oily aromatic liquid. This balsamic resin is extracted by cutting deeply into the trunks of trees that grow primarily in Indonesia and Thailand.

benzophenone-2—a sunscreen chemical with UV-absorbing properties.

benzophenone-3 (AKA oxybenzone)—a sunscreen chemical. It is an oil-soluble UV absorber with absorption rates within the UVA and UVB peak ranges. Its popularity in sunscreen formulations is increasing as manufacturers become more concerned with potential safety problems associated with more traditional sunscreen chemicals.

benzophenone-4 (AKA sulisobenzone)—an FDA-approved sunscreen chemical with UVA absorbing properties and an approved usage level of 5–10%. Also considered an antiphoto-oxidant.

benzophenone-8 (AKA dioxybenzone)—an FDA-approved sunscreen chemical with UVA absorption capabilities.

benzoyl peroxide—an antibacteria ingredient commonly used in acne treatments. It functions by forcing an oxidant (peroxide in this case) into the pilosebaceous orifice where it releases oxygen, thereby diminishing the *P. acnes* population. This reduces the level of free fatty acids and the level of skin infection. Benzoyl peroxide may cause skin irritation to people with sensitive skin. As a topical retinoid it also may cause dryness, irritation, allergic contact dermatitis, and phototoxicity.

benzyl alcohol—a preservative against bacteria used in concentrations of 1.0–3.0%. It can cause skin irritation.

benzylidene camphor (AKA 3-benzylidene camphor)—used as a UVB sunscreen.

benzyl laurate—an emollient ester that is easily emulsified and leaves the skin feeling silky. It is nontoxic, nonirritating, nonviscous and nonoily. It also reduces the oiliness of mineral oil and solubilizes sunscreen actives.

bergamot oil (*Citrus bergamia, Monarda didyma*)—considered an antiseptic and bacterial growth inhibitor. It is also considered good for oily and acne skin and for seborrheic conditions. Sun exposure after applying pure bergamot oil or a compound with a high bergamot oil concentration to the skin may cause hyperpigmentation and a skin rash. When used in perfumes its photosensitizing properties are responsible for the hyperpigmentation seen behind the ear and on the neck area near the ear. The oil extracted from the rind of citrus fruits is referred to as bergamot orange. Regular bergamot is from the monarda plant of which there are several varieties.

beta-carotene—a major constituent of carrot oil. It has known antioxidant and photoprotection properties and is also used as a yellow-orange color additive. Its strong color and tendency to stain the skin often limits its use. While colorless versions are now becoming available to cosmetic formulators the specific value of these has not yet been determined. *See also* carotene.

beta-glucan—*see* glucans; polyglucan.

18 beta-glycerrhentinic acid (AKA glycyrrhetic acid)—a triterpenic acid credited with anti-inflammatory, decongestant, and redness-reducing properties. It can also act as an epithelial regenerator. Used effectively in milks, creams, and gels for the treatment of sensitive skins. Obtained from the hydrolysis of glycyrrhizic acid. *See also* glycyrrhizic acid.

betaine—a surfactant and an excellent conditioner, viscosity builder, and foam booster. It is found mostly in skin cleansers, shampoos, and bath products.

betony extract *(Stachys officinalis)*—traditionally used in dermatological disorders as a soothing and anti-itching treatment. It is recommended for problem skin.

BHA (AKA butylated hydroxyanisole)—a preservative with antioxidant capabilities.

BHT (AKA butylated hydroxytoluene)—a toluene-based preservative with antioxidant properties. Toluene-based ingredients are rarely used in skin care cosmetics as toluene is not a good product base for the skin.

bioflavonoid—a plant derivative with therapeutic attributes. It has antioxidant properties that allow it to absorb oxygen radicals that may cause skin oxidation, and antimicrobial activity that may aid in anti-inflammatory capabilities against microbially caused skin irritations. An ingredient listing of this sort fails to identify the specific botanical(s) involved and may then refer to a group of compounds.

biological serum—considered a good carrier of essential fatty acids to the epidermal cells. It is also recommended as a cell growth factor in cultures. It is reported that when biological serum is applied to the skin, it helps increase the epidermal cell renewal rate. Biological serum is the fluid portion that remains after removal of fibrin clots and blood cells. It may contain about 11% protein.

Biophytex—a manufacturer's name for a combination of plant extracts including butchersbroom, horse chestnut, and Indian water nave. Reported to have calming, desensitizing, and minor healing properties.

biotin (AKA biotine; vitamin H)—some cosmetic manufacturers claim biotin has healing properties and as such is a good ingredient for acne skin. A deficiency of this vitamin has been associated with greasy scalp and baldness. Its deficiency in humans is considered extremely rare, and the value of external application via cosmetic products is questionable.

biotine—*see* biotin.

birch (*Betula* sp.)—actual clinical data is scant in substantiating its therapeutic effects as well as those of its derivatives. Birch and birch derivatives have been described as astringent, antiseptic, softening, and circulation stimulating and they are believed to have curative properties in cases of skin diseases. In folklore, birch has been used for its healing effects on rashes and in cases of hair loss. Birch's important constituents include glanonoids, hyperoside, tannin, saponins, and quercetin. Even though some manufacturers list this ingredient as simply "birch," a proper description should be more specific, i.e., birch bark extract, birch leaf extract, or birch sap. *See also* birch bark extract.

birch bark extract—described as having anti-irritant and antiseptic properties with effectiveness in acne treatment and sunburn products, soothing lotions, and aftershaves. The oil is astringent and is mainly used for its curative effects, especially in cases of acne and eczema. In folkloric medicine, birch bark extract was considered good for bathing skin eruptions. Destructive distillation of the bark's white epidermis yields an empyreumatic oil, known as oil of birch tar, *Oleum rusci,* or dagget. This is a thick, bituminous, brownish black liquid with a pungent, balsamic odor. It contains a high percentage of methylsalicilate, creosol, and guaiacol. It is almost identical to wintergreen oil.

birch leaf extract—believed to have antiseptic and astringent properties and to help heal skin irritations. It is used in traditional medicine for skin rashes. The leaves, which have a peculiar, aromatic, yet agreeable odor and a bitter taste, secrete a resinous substance with acid properties. They contain flavonoids, tannins, and essential oils.

birch sap—claimed to drain water.

bisabolol—a botanical claimed to be anti-inflammatory and soothing. It is derived from chamomile and/or yarrow.

bismuth oxychloride—an inorganic color additive. It is used mostly in makeup manufacturing and rarely in skin care formulations. It may also be used for pearlization in cosmetics.

bitter almond extract—an emollient and a carrier, it may cause irritation and negative skin reactions. *See also* almond oil, bitter.

bitter orange extract *(Citrus aurantium)*—a botanical credited with soothing properties. It is obtained from the peel of bitter oranges, and it has a more delicate fragrance than sweet orange. *See also* orange extract.

black catechu—*see* acacia.

black currant extract *(Ribes nigrum)*—its therapeutic uses are not clear, though some report it to be anti-inflammatory. The whole plant may be used, including the fruit, leaves, bark, and roots.

black currant seed oil—may be an effective ingredient for enhancing the skin's ability to develop normal barrier functions and the protective effect of the corneum layer. Black currant seed oil contains fatty, linoleic, and linolenic acids. When applied to dry skin it may increase the skin's own content of these previously lacking components.

black pepper oil—its cosmetic application is unclear, though it may be used on skin inflammations and superficial wounds. This oil is obtained from a small-grain black pepper shrub found primarily in the hilly parts of Jamaica.

black tang—*see* seaweed extract.

black tea extract—*see* tea extract.

black walnut extract—an antiseptic, noncomedogenic raw material. *See also* walnut.

blackberry extract *(Rubus villosus)*—regarded as excellent for its astringent and tonic properties due to the high tannin content of the root bark and the leaves. The leaf extract can be beneficially used for acne conditions.

bladderwrack—*see* seaweed extract.

blessed thistle extract (AKA holy thistle)—tonic and stimulating properties have been attributed to this herb. It is an effective extract for problem skin. In antiquity, it was felt that this plant aided in the healing of skin sores and had the ability to reduce itching. Blessed thistle contains a volatile oil and a bitter, crystalline neutral body called Cnicin, said to be analogous to salicin in its properties. One of many varieties of thistle.

bloodroot—*see* tetterwort extract.

blue centaury extract—*see* cornflower extract.

***bois de rose* oil**—a fragrance with a light camphor scent. This essential oil is obtained via steam distillation of the chipped wood from the tropical rosewood tree. *Bois de rose* oil has no known toxicity.

borage extract *(Borago officinalis)* (AKA borago)—its topical application is described as anti inflammatory. It is beneficial for sensitive skin and allergic reactions. Borage contains potassium and calcium, combined with mineral acids. This is a hardy annual plant of which the leaves and, to a lesser degree, the flowers are used.

borage oil—*see* borage extract.

boric acid—an effective preservative against yeast. It is used in concentrations of 0.01–1.0% and has fair to good antiseptic properties. The use of boric acid in cosmetic preparations is no longer very popular. Boric acid is prepared from sulfuric acid and natural borax. It can cause skin rashes and irritation if used in high concentrations.

borneol—utilized in perfumery for its peppery odor. Borneol is a naturally occurring substance found in coriander, ginger oil, oil of lime, rosemary, strawberries, thyme, citronella, and nutmeg. Its toxicity is similar to that of camphor. *See also* camphor.

bovine amniotic fluid—*see* amniotic fluid.

bovine liver extract—one of many available biologicals of animal origin. *See also* protein.

bovine serum—*see* bovine serum albumin.

bovine serum albumin—reported to be a good carrier of fatty acids to the epidermic cells and, in combination with certain other ingredients it may help increase the epidermal cell renewal rate. It is used in preparations designed for temporary wrinkle removal.

bovine spleen extract—reported to improve oxygenation and the elimination of cell waste.

brain extract—contributes to a formulation's ability to assist in the rapid repair of the skin's permeability barrier. It functions by positioning itself in the intercorneocyte spaces of the corneum layer, thereby improving the composition of intercellular cement. This bovine extract is rich in cephalin, a substance found in the body, especially the brain and spinal cord.

bran extract—used in peels and scrubs for its mild abrasive qualities.

Brazilian babassu nut oil—*see* babassu oil.

brewer's yeast—*see* yeast.

brewing grain extracts—said to be anti-inflammatory with some anti-irritant properties. Brewing grain extracts are reported to inhibit certain types or erythema, relieve skin itching, and provide an antimycotic effect. The grains include barley and wheat.

British gum—*see* dextrin.

2-bromo-2 nitro-1,3 propane diol—a preservative. It is effective against a broad range of microorganisms but it performs better against fungi and yeast. It becomes inactive in sulfur-containing formulas. Used in concentrations of 0.01–0.1% it is nontoxic, nonirritating, and nonsensitizing to humans. Safe as a cosmetic ingredient up to and including 0.1% concentrations except under circumstances where its reaction with amines and amides can result in the formation of nitrosamines or nitrosamides. It has a slightly higher than moderate sensitizing potential in leave-on cosmetic preparations. Unstable at high temperatures.

brown seaweed—*see* seaweed.

buckthorn—*see* cascara sagrada extract.

burdock—*see* burdock root extract.

burdock root extract *(Arctium lappa)*—credited with antibacterial and antifungal properties and an apparent ability to help regulate/normalize oil production. Traditionally used in the treatment of mild acne conditions. When applied externally as a compress burdock leaves are considered highly effective for relieving bruises and inflammation. Burdock's constituents include inulin, mucilage, sugar, a crystalline glucoside called lappin, fixed and volatile oils, and some tannic acid. Extracts from the fruit (commonly though mistakenly referred to as the seeds) are also considered beneficial for chronic skin diseases. The dried root and root extract are the official therapeutic segments of burdock.

Burow's solution—*see* aluminum acetate solution.

butchersbroom extract *(Ruscus aculeatus)*—no clear benefit for skin care application has been attributed to this botanical. Some sources cite it as having slimming and anticellulite effects as well as diuretic and anti-itching properties. Butchersbroom is a low, shrubby evergreen plant of which the herb and the root are used.

butyl oleate—an ester of butyl alcohol and oleic acid with lubricant, moisturizer, and emollient properties.

butyl paraben—a preservative with little sensitizing effect against fungi and yeast. It is generally used in combination with other preservatives to increase the preservative activity spectrum. Butyl paraben is only effective in the acid pH range. *See also* parabens.

butyl stearate—a stearic acid used in very small quantities in cosmetic preparations as an emulsifier for creams and lotions. It has been shown to cause allergic reactions.

butylated hydroxyanisole—*see* BHA.

butylated hydroxytoluene—*see* BHT.

butyldiadipate—an emollient and pH-adjusting agent with good penetrating properties.

butylene glycol—a solvent with good antimicrobial action. It enhances the preservative activity of parabens.

1,3 butylene glycol—a solvent and viscosity-decreasing agent commonly used in cosmetic and toiletry preparations.

butylmethoxy dibenzoylmethane—considered a highly efficient UVA sunscreen. Not used by U.S. sunscreen manufacturers because it is not on the FDA's Category I list.

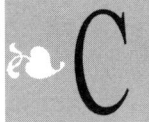

cactus extract—an emulsifier for creams and lotions that, as an active substance, is described as good for sunburns and other minor burns, insect bites, skin irritations, swelling, and inflammation. It has been used in folklore medicine for dropsy. Its sticky, gelatinous quality makes it valuable for face masks, particularly the clear, peel-off types. The main constituents of cactus include cactin, flavonoids, amino acids, and polysaccharides.

caffeine—although incorporated into some cosmetic formulations, its current use in cosmetics has not been identified. This bitter-tasting, odorless white powder occurs naturally in coffee, cola, guarna paste, kola nuts, and tea. Caffeine is obtained as a by-product of decaffeinated coffee.

cajeput oil *(Melaleuca leucadendron)* (AKA eucalyptol)—used externally for psoriasis and other skin problems. It has healing, antiseptic, stimulating, and mildly counterirritant properties. The principal constituent of this oil is cineol, which averages 45–55%. Also present is solid terpineol as well as several aldehydes such as valeric, butyric, and benzoic. *See also* eucalyptus oil.

calamine—has mildly astringent and cooling qualities and is particularly useful for sunburned or irritated skin. Calamine is a mineral solution consisting primarily of zinc oxide with the addition of approximately 0.5% ferric oxide.

calamint *(Calamintha officinalis)* (AKA calamintha)—considered to reduce bruising. Calamint contains a camphoraceous, volatile, stimulating oil in common with the other mints. Obtained from a bushy plant closely related to the thyme family and ground ivy.

calamintha—*see* calamint.

calcium alginate—used as a visual accent in cosmetics. This is an alginate gel impregnated with an oily core material that can be pigmented or neutral in color.

calcium chloride—a compound that helps improve the reaction among certain ingredients used in cosmetic formulations. This inorganic salt is now rarely used in skin care products and is being replaced with potassium chloride.

calcium hydroxide—an inorganic base employed as a topical astringent and alkali in solutions or lotions. It can burn the skin and eyes.

calcium pantothenate—used as an emollient and to enrich creams and lotions in hair care preparations. This is the calcium salt of pantothenic acid found in liver, rice, bran, and molasses. It is also found in large amounts in royal jelly.

calcium thioglycolate—used almost exclusively in depilatory creams and hair products, this is a calcium salt of thioglycolic acid. It may cause skin irritation.

calendula extract *(Calendula officinalis)* (AKA marigold)—an emollient said to have healing, soothing, antiseptic, anti-itching, and anti-inflammatory properties. It can be effectively used in cases of oily and/or delicate skin as well as for acne. The extract is obtained from the calendula blossom. *See also* marigold extract.

calendula hydrolysates—a calendula derivative. *See also* calendula extract.

calf serum—*see* bovine serum.

calfskin extract—an oil-soluble extract of bovine skin. *See also* protein.

camellia oil—used as a nongreasy emollient for skin care products. Camellia oil plays an important role in antioxidation as a result of its high content of oleic acid. Derived from the seeds of *Thea sasanqua nois*.

camphor *(Cinnamomum camphora)*—credited with anesthetic, anti-inflammatory, antiseptic, astringent, cooling, and refreshing properties and thought to be slightly stimulating to the blood circulation and function. Once absorbed by the subcutaneous tissue, it combines in the body with glucoronic acid and in this condition is voided by the urine. Camphor is effective for oily and acne skin treatment and has a scent similar to eucalyptus. In high concentrations it can be an irritant and numb the peripheral sensory nerves. Natural camphor is derived from an evergreen tree indigenous to the Orient, though now its synthetic substitute is often used.

camphor oil—*see* camphor.

candelilla wax—binds oils and waxes and gives body to a formulation. Obtained from candelilla plants.

candlenut—*see* kukui nut oil.

canola oil—has good emolliency and lubricity. Canola oil is a rapeseed oil extract considered to be a natural replacement for mineral oil.

caprylic/capric triglyceride (AKA Tricaprylin)—an emollient with good spreading properties. It promotes penetration and does not leave visible traces of grease on the skin. It is effectively used in creams, lotions, and oil formulations.

caprylol collagen amino acids—a liquid with an antiacne effect. *See also* amino acid; collagen.

capryloyl collagenic acid—this lipoamino acid is found to have similar antibacterial properties as benzoyl peroxide when tested against *S. aureus, S. epidermidis,* and *P. acnes* bacterias. Test results show it to be most effective and helpful in treating mild cases of acne vulgaris, though it demonstrates some positive results against moderate and severe acne cases as well. Although it reduces inflammatory lesions, it does not affect comedones and cysts. When treatment is suspended there is a mild relapse of the acne lesions.

caprylyl/capryl glucoside—a surfactant used in cleansing preparations, primarily shampoos.

caramel—used as a coloring agent. It provides products with a slight touch of brown. Some sources also state that it acts as a soothing agent in some skin care preparations. Caramel is a concentrated solution obtained from heating sugar or glucose solutions.

caraway oil *(Carum carvi)*—a carrier oil credited with the ability to remove bruises and believed to have tissue- regenerating properties. It is said to be beneficial for acne and oily skin. Caraway is a member of the group of aromatic, umbelliferous plants, such as anise, cumin, dill, and fennel, characterized by carminative properties. Carvene (also found in dill and cumin oils), and an oxygenated oil, and carvol are the principal constituents of caraway oil. Caraway oil is obtained from the distillation of the seeds and may cause allergic reactions and skin irritation.

carbocysteine—an amino acid used in cosmetic formulations. *See also* amino acid.

carbomer 934, 940, 941, 980, 981—these high-molecular-weight cross-linked polymers are used as thickening and suspending agents and emulsion stabilizers in cosmetic formulations. They are often used with triethanolamine, sodium hydroxide, or other alkaline compounds to cross-link the polymer. White, slightly acidic powders, carbomers react with fat particles to form thick stable emulsions of oils in water.

Carbopol—a trade name for carbomer. *See also* carbomer.

carboxyethy-γ-aminobutyric acid—described as an ingredient promoting cellular growth. May be used in antiaging preparations.

carboxymethyl cellulose (AKA cellulose gum)—a thickener like Carbopol. Used in cosmetic formulations when a reactant (potassium chloride in the case of Carbopol) is not required or desired. Often used in bath preparations, beauty masks, hand creams, and shampoos. It is considered a noncomedogenic raw material.

carboxymethyl chitin—considered to be one of the best new moisturizing ingredients. Carboxymethyl chitin is derived from the exoskeleton of shrimp and crab. *See also* chitin.

carboxypolymethylene—*see* carbomer.

carboxyvinyl polymer—provides viscosity and is suitable for both thickening and stabilizing emulsions or dispersions in cosmetics. Its incorporation into cosmetic formulations results in very clear gel preparations. A synthetic resin.

cardamom oil *(Elettaria cardamomum)*—credited with antiseptic, stimulating, and deodorant properties. This is a large perennial herb that yields cardamom seeds containing volatile oil, fixed oil, salt of potassium, a coloring principle, starch, nitrogenous mucilage, ligneous fiber, an acrid resin, and ash. The volatile oil contains terpenes, terpineol, and cineol.

carmellia seed powder—an ingredient from the Orient currently in vogue for its abrasive action.

carmine—a crimson pigment. This is the aluminum lake of the coloring agent cochineal, which is a natural pigment derived from the dried female insect *Coccus cacti*. Carmine may cause allergic reactions.

carnauba wax—used to firm and texturize cosmetic preparations and give them a less fluid consistency. Carnauba wax also forms a protective layer on the skin's surface. It has the highest melting point among natural plant waxes and does not usually cause allergic reactions. This wax is obtained from leaves and leaf buds of the Brazilian wax palm.

carnitine—a skin-conditioning agent, surfactant, and formulation viscosity-increasing substance. Carnitine is used primarily in hand and body preparations.

carob extract *(Jacaranda procera, Caroba balsam)*—its botanical property is reported as anti-infectious. In the small leaves—carob extract's source—caroborelinic acid, carobic acid, steocarobic acid, carobon, and carobin have been found.

carotene—used to provide a red-orange color in cosmetic formulations. It is the primary yellow coloring component of butter, carrots, and egg yolk. Carotene is found in plants as well as many animal tissues. Beta-carotene is an effective antioxidant. *See also* beta-carotene.

carotene oil—a red-orange colored oil containing carotene. A carrot extract.

carrageen extract *(Chondrus crispus)* (AKA Irish moss)—a very common thickener that, in its sodium salt form, has jellifying properties. Carrageen is a polysaccharide of red algae origin with a seaweedlike odor and is considered nontoxic. *See also* seaweed extract.

carreghane extract (AKA red algae)—*see* seaweed extract.

carrot extract *(Daucus carota)*—there are some indications that, when obtained from carrot leaves, the extract may have cleansing and healing properties due to its strong antiseptic qualities. The root contains no less than 89% water. The juice also contains sugar, a little starch, extractine gluten, albumen, volatile oil, vegetable jelly or pectin, saline matter, malic acid, and carotin. Carrot's botanical properties depend on its volatile oil.

carrot oil—used since the sixteenth century for skin diseases due to its believed cleansing, depurative, and draining properties. This carotene-rich emollient has been indicated for acne skin conditions, dermatitis, skin irritation, skin rashes, and wrinkles. Derived from the carrot root.

carrot oleoresin—has good conditioning properties. This ingredient is found more often in hair care products.

cascara sagrada extract *(Rhamnus purshiana)* (AKA buckthorn; sacred bark)—used to add a skin-soothing factor in lotions and creams. The assertion has been made that the bark contains glucosides. The extract is prepared from this shrub's bark.

casein amino acids—hydrolyzed milk protein. Used as an emulsifier in many cosmetics. It also binds water for moisturization. *See also* amino acids.

castor oil—a highly emollient carrier oil that penetrates the skin easily, leaving it soft and supple. It also serves to bind the different ingredients of a cosmetic formulation together. Its unpleasant odor makes it difficult to use in cosmetics. Castor oil is high in glycerin esters of ricinoleic acid. It is rarely, if ever, associated with irritation of the skin or allergic reactions. Obtained through cold-pressing from seeds or beans of the *Ricinus communis* (castor oil) plant. Impure castor oil may cause irritation as the seeds contain a toxic substance that is eliminated during processing.

caviar—*see* roe extract.

cedar—*see* cedarwood oil.

cedarwood oil *(Thuja occidentalis)* (AKA cedar; thuja)— credited with antiseptic, sedative, and astringent properties. This clear oil is also valuable for use on skin eruptions and to relieve itching. It is good for acne and oily skin and could be helpful in cases of dermatitis, eczema, and psoriasis. It is used as a fixative in fragrances because it blends well with other oils. Two types of cedarwood oil exist: Atlas cedarwood oil from Morocco *(Cedrus atlantica)* and one derived from the *Juniperus virginiana* (or red cedar) that is actually a juniper of the United States (its oil, however, is very similar to true cedarwood). The oil may cause skin irritation when used in high concentrations. Cedarwood oil is obtained from recently dried, leafy, young twigs.

cell cytoplasm derivative—a functional fraction of mushroom extract.

cellular extracts—help repair the skin. *See also* amniotic fluid; bovine serum albumin; protein.

cellular protein—*see* protein.

cellulose—a thickener and an emulsifier. Obtained from plants.

cellulose (microcrystalline)—used as an emulsifier in cosmetic creams. It is the chief constituent of plant fiber.

cellulose fiber—used as a thickener, suspending agent, and binder.

cellulose gum—a thickener and an emulsifier equivalent to cellulose fiber. It is resistant to bacterial decomposition and provides a product with uniform viscosity. Constituents are any of several fibrous substances consisting of the chief part of a plant's cell walls. *See also* carboxymethyl cellulose.

ceramides—act primarily in the uppermost skin layer, affecting the intercellular spaces of the corneum layer where they form a protective barrier and reduce the natural transepidermal water loss of the skin. Ceramides repair the corneum layer in cases of dry skin, improve skin hydration, and increase the feeling of softness. They are naturally present in the skin, forming an integral part of the intercellular membrane network. Natural ceramides are obtained from animals and plants. However, regardless of their source, it is very difficult to isolate the types of highly pure ceramides necessary for cosmetics. In addition, ceramides identical to those found in nature are hard to synthesize, making ceramides expensive raw materials of limited application in the cosmetic industry.

cereal lipoplastidins—coconut oil that has been mixed with a number of cereal grain extracts such as rice, bran, and/or oat.

cereal germ oil—a carrier.

cereal seed oils—a carrier.

cerebrosides—their incorporation into skin care products (many times under the name of ceramides) appears to

109

greatly improve the look and texture of the skin surface. Research studies indicate that cerebrosides accumulate within the corneum layer, repairing damaged segments, improving cellular organization, and increasing the number of corneum layers. In the skin they are produced in basal epidermal cells and secreted externally, where they form protective coatings around the viable cells. As the corneum layer keratinizes, the cerebrosides are, in part, hydrolyzed to yield ceramides. Cerebrosides originally were obtained as an extract of bovine or swine crude brain. Researchers have been working to obtain cerebrosides from plants such as *Malvaceae* and pearl millet, both with reasonable amounts of glycolipids.

ceresin—incorporated into skin care formulations in order to regulate the viscosity, suspension properties, and overall stability of a preparation. Used in protective creams as a beeswax and paraffin substitute. This white to yellow waxy mixture of hydrocarbons is obtained by the purification of ozokerite. Ceresin is a waxy material that may cause allergic reactions.

ceresin wax (AKA ceresin)—a thickener and a binder with noncomedogenic properties. *See also* ceresin.

ceteareth—used as an emollient, emulsifier, antifoam agent, and lubricant in cosmetic formulations. Ceteareth is obtained from a combination of cetyl alcohol and stearyl alcohol.

ceteareth 4—an emulsifier. The polyethylene glycol ether of cetearyl alcohol.

ceteareth 12—an emulsifier.

ceteareth 19—an emulsifier.

ceteareth 20—a good solubilizer and emulsifier.

ceteareth 30—an emulsifier and solubilizing agent.

cetearyl alcohol (AKA cetostearyl alcohol)—an emulsifying and stabilizing wax produced from the reduction of plant oils and natural waxes. Also used as an emollient and to give high viscosity to a finished product. Cetearyl alcohol is a mixture of fatty alcohols consisting primarily of cetyl and stearyl alcohols.

cetearyl glucoside—an emulsifying substance.

cetearyl isononandate—an emollient with a high hydrophobic effect.

cetearyl octanoate—an emollient. This ingredient can be either a palm kernel or coconut derivative and has a high degree of water repellency. It is used in noncomedogenic moisturizers. In nature it occurs on the feathers of water birds.

cetearyl palmitate—when incorporated into a skin care product it leaves the skin with a velvety feel. This ingredient is used as a replacement for spermaceti wax.

ceteth—used as a surface active agent in cosmetics. A ceteth is a compound of derivatives of cetyl, lauryl, stearyl, and oleyl alcohols mixed with ethylene oxide.

ceteth 20—an emulsifier for oil-in-water creams and lotions.

cetostearyl alcohol—*see* cetearyl alcohol.

cetrimonium bromide —*see* cetyl trimethylammonium bromide.

cetyl alcohol—an emollient, emulsifier, and thickener produced from palm oil or spermaceti. It is also found in coconut and other vegetable oils and is made synthetically. Considered by some sources to be a noncomedogenic material.

cetyl alcohol 40—a preservative and carrier similar to cetyl alcohol.

cetyl dimethicone—an emollient and occlusive skin-conditioning agent based on silicones.

cetyl dimethicone copolyol—an emulsifier and emollient used in cosmetic preparations to form water-in-oil emulsions that have viscosity but also rub out easily. These types of preparations are used in sunscreen formulations where good spreadability and waterproofing are valued characteristics. Used in moisturizers, these emulsions provide a good moisture barrier and reduce the speed of transepidermal water loss.

cetyl esters—used in formulations to give body to emulsions. They are also formulation stabilizers and thickeners. Cetyl esters are generally indistinguishable from natural spermaceti wax in terms of composition and properties. Cetyl esters are made from a combination of various fatty esters with cetyl palmitate.

cetyl palmitate (AKA synthetic spermaceti)—its chemical structure is the same as whale spermaceti. It may be used to thicken, produce viscose emulsions, give stability, and add texture to emulsions. It is similar to cetearyl palmitate.

cetyl phosphate—a mild emulsifier with a low irritancy potential.

cetyl ricinoleate—an emollient and emulsion stabilizer considered to be a noncomedogenic ester.

cetyl trimethylammonium bromide (AKA cetrimonium bromide)—a cosmetic bioside and an emulsifying agent. A quaternary ammonium salt.

chamomile extract *(Anthemis nobilis* and *Matricaria chamomilla)*—has clinically proven anti-inflammatory and repairer properties. It is also considered bactericidal, anti-itching, soothing, antiseptic, purifying, refreshing, and hypoallergenic with ability to neutralize skin irritants. There are various forms of chamomile, including Roman chamomile *(Anthemis nobilis)* and German chamomile *(Matricaria chamomilla)*. German chamomile tends to be more potent than Roman due to its higher azulene content. Active constituents include azulene, bisabolol, and phytosterol. The chamomile plant is aromatic, and its flower heads are used to obtain aqueous-alcoholic extracts and the blue chamomile oil. Chamomile is considered a noncomedogenic raw material and can be beneficially used in aftershaves and eye treatment preparations as well as products for dry skin.

chamomile oil—considered a capillarian wall constrictor, anti-allergenic agent, antiseptic, cooling, analgesic, and healing. It has been found to be good for treating burns and skin inflammations as well as dermatitis. Chamomile oil also has emollient properties. It is good for use with acne, dry, or supersensitive skin. The active principles are a pale blue volatile oil (which can turn yellow with keeping), a little anthemic acid, tannic acid, and a glucoside. The volatile oil obtained through distillation is lost in the preparation of the extract. The whole plant is odoriferous and of value, but the flowerheads are primarily credited with therapeutic benefits. Since the chief botanical virtue of the plant lies in the central disk of the yellow florets and in the cultivated double form of the white florets, it is considered that the botanical properties of the single, wild chamomile are the most powerful.

chamomile flower oil—*see* chamomile oil.

chaulmoogra oil *(Taraktogenos kurzii)*—a soothing and anti-inflammatory oil. It is considered by some to be healing, with good application in acne cases. It contains chaulmoogric acid and palmitic acid. Its fatty oil constituent has been found to yield glycerol, a very small quantity of phytosterol, and a mixture of fatty acids. Chaulmoogra oil can be irritating and have an unpleasant odor. It is obtained from the seeds of *Taraktogenos kurzii.*

chestnut extract *(Castanea sativa)*—due to its high tannin content the extract from the bark is claimed to have astringent effect when applied topically.

China clay—*see* kaolin.

Chinese angelica root—*see* angelica.

chitin (AKA chitine)—a moisture retainer and film-forming agent. This is a polysaccharide from the exoskeletons of gastropods such as shrimp and crab. Chitosa, the decarboxylated form of chitin, holds water without tackiness.

chitine—*see* chitin.

chitosan—forms a film on the skin's surface and aids in moisture retention. This ingredient enhances liposome stability through chemical interactions.

chlorhexidine—used as a topical antiseptic and as a skin-sterilizing agent in liquid cosmetics. It is strongly alkaline and may cause irritation.

chlorhexidine digluconate—a preservative generally used in concentrations of 0.01–0.1% to protect against bacteria. It is unstable at high temperatures. Chlorhexidine digluconate is more widely used in Europe than in the United States. *See also* chlorhexidine.

5 chloro-2 methyl-4 isothiazolin 3 one and 2-methyl 4 5-hydroxy-2-styryl-4-pyrones — a skin-lightening agent due to its ability to inhibit melanin formation. It is stable and nonirritating to the skin.

chlorophenesin—a preservative.

chlorophyll—used as a natural coloring agent. It is credited with skin-soothing and healing properties and has a mild deodorizing effect. Its healing and soothing values are attributed to its phytol content. Chlorophyll is the green coloring matter found in all living plants and seen in plant leaves.

chlorophyllin copper complex—a color additive obtained from chlorophyll. *See also* chlorophyll.

chloroxyethanol—a preservative with low sensitizing potential.

cholesteric esters — a cholesterol derivative. *See also* cholesterol.

cholesterol—a moisturizer and emollient that acts as a powerful emulsifier in water-in-oil systems. Cholesterol is a fatlike substance found in plant and animal cells. It is also present in the secretion of the sebaceous glands and therefore is a component of the fat on the skin's surface. Considered a noncomedogenic raw material. It may sometimes be obtained from sheep's wool wax.

choleth 24—an emulsifying agent considered a noncomedogenic raw material. It is often employed for its moisturizing action. A polyethylene glycol ether of cholesterol.

chondroitin sulfate—reported to increase water-binding properties when used with hydrolyzed protein and to enhance the moisturizing effects of creams and lotions.

In the skin, chondroitin sulfate is a component of the natural glycosaminoglycans.

Chondrus crispus **extract** (AKA brown seaweed)—*see* seaweed extract.

chromium compounds—these are oxides used primarily for green eye shadows and greenish mascaras. Chromium compounds may cause allergic reactions when applied to the skin.

chromium hydroxide green—a color additive used primarily in makeup preparations. *See also* chromium compounds.

chromium oxide green—a color additive used primarily in makeup preparations. *See also* chromium compounds.

cinchena—*see* cinchona extract.

cinchona extract *(Cinchona ledgeriana)* (AKA cinchena; quinquina)—a major source of quinine. Cinchona extract has long been known for its tonic, antiseptic, and astringent properties. It has also been commonly used as a remedy for malaria and fever in tropical areas. It is obtained from the bark of various Latin American plant species belonging to the *Linnaean* genus. If used in large quantities, cinchona will cause headaches and nausea in those allergic to it.

cinnamic acid—has sunscreen capabilities. Some manufacturers use it to replace PABA due to its lower allergic and phototoxic reaction incidence. Cinnamic acid is found in cinnamon leaves and cocoa leaves and is an essential oil of certain mushrooms. It may cause allergic skin rashes.

cinnamon oil *(Cinnamomum zeylanicum)*—said to have a soothing effect on the skin. It can also be used for fragrance. Widely recognized for its tonic and antiseptic properties, cinnamon oil is very important in traditional pharmacopoeia. It is obtained from distillation of the plant's leaves. It can cause irritation if used in high doses.

cinnamon bark oil—has similar properties to those of cinnamon oil, but this distillation of the plant's bark is considered of much higher quality than extractions from leaves. Use in high doses or in high concentrations could produce skin irritations. *See also* cinnamon oil.

cinoxate (AKA 2-hydroxy-p-methoxycinnamate)—an FDA-approved sunscreen chemical with an approved usage level of 1–3%. *See also* cinnamic acid.

cinquefoil extract *(Potentilla anserina)* (AKA five leaf grass; silverweed)—an astringent ingredient incorporated into formulations for its anti-inflammatory and healing properties. It can be of value for problem skin. Cinquefoil is a creeping plant with large yellow flowers. The extract is obtained from the herb and root of the plant.

citric acid—has astringent and antioxidant properties. It can also be used as a preservative with a low sensitizing potential. It is not usually irritating to normal skin, but it can cause burning and redness when applied to chapped, cracked, or otherwise inflamed skin. Derived from citrus fruits.

citric oils—refers to one or a combination of oils from citrus fruits such as orange oil, lemon oil, grapefruit oil, etc.

citronella java oil—antiseptic and widely used in soaps and deodorizers. It may also have insect repellent properties. This herb distillation may cause a skin rash when used in cosmetics.

clary sage oil *(Salvia sclarea)* (AKA sclary sage oil)—could be beneficial in products designed for use around the eyes due to its soothing and anti-inflammatory properties. Its fragrance may have aromatherapeutic value such as promoting cell regeneration for normal, dry, and sensitive skin types.

clay—as a general ingredient category, it may include bentonite, beegum, and China clay. This mineral is used as a clarifying agent in liquids, as an emollient, and as a poultice. It can also serve as a color component in face powders, face masks, body powders, and makeup foundations. It does not cause skin allergies.

clay-earth—*see* clay.

clay sediments—*see* clay.

cleavers extract *(Galium aparine)*—said to be useful in treating eczema and spots. Cleavers extract is recommended for normal to dry skins.

clematis—the extract from the plant's roots and stems has anti-inflammatory action, but the leaves and the flowers, when crushed, irritate the eyes and, when applied to the skin, produce inflammation. Clematis is a perennial plant.

climbing ivy extract—*see* ivy.

clove oil *(Caryophyllus aromaticus, Syzygium aromaticum)*—considered a powerful antiseptic and cicatrizant with a strong germicidal effect. This oil was traditionally used to clean small wounds. Clove oil may cause strong skin irritation when used in high concentrations, although in diluted forms it is generally harmless. This oil is obtained from stems and leaves of a small evergreen tree.

clove bud oil—has similar properties to clove oil. However, the distillates from dried buds are considered of higher quality than the ones obtained from the stems and leaves.

Clove oil derived from the plant's leaves is sometimes used to adulterate the oil obtained from the bud.

clover extract (*Trifolium* sp.)—the fluid extract is used as an antispasmodic. A short-lived perennial plant, clover produces abundant blossoms that are used in herbal oils and extracts.

clover blossom extract—credited with astringent properties. *See also* clover.

club moss extract (*Lycopodium clavatum*)—the spores of club moss have traditionally been used as an external dusting powder for various skin diseases and wounded surfaces. The tops of the plants are cut as the spikes approach maturity, and the powder is shaken out and separated with a sieve. Commercially used spores are probably also derived from additional moss species.

cocamide DEA—a thickener and viscosity builder for cosmetic surfactant systems. It is added to liquid cleansers of the lauryl sulfate variety to help stabilize the lather and improve foam formation.

cocamidopropyl PG-dimonium chloride phosphate—an antimicrobial and antifungal that is very mild to the skin. *See also* coconut oil.

cocamidopropyl betaine—a surfactant derived from a coconut oil salt. It is particularly effective in shampoos, foam baths, shower foams, and other preparations where a high, creamy foam and good skin tolerance are desired. *See also* coconut oil.

cocoa butter—softens and lubricates the skin. This yellowish vegetal fat is solid at room temperature but liquifies below body temperature, and is frequently used in lip balms and massage creams due to its favorable melting point. Cocoa butter is considered comedogenic and may cause allergic reactions.

coco-caprylate/caprate—a light and cosmetically elegant emollient obtained from vegetable sources.

cocoamidopropylamine oxide—a conditioner, viscosity builder and foam booster. Derived from coconut oil.

cocoampho carboxyglycinate—used as a skin softener and lubricant and commonly incorporated into soaps and creams. It is a solid fat from cocoa plant seeds.

coconut oil—used as a cream base. A raw material in soaps, ointments, massage creams, and in sunscreen formulations. Soft white or slightly yellow in color and semisolid in consistency, coconut oil is a grouping of primarily short-chain fatty acids bonded with glycerin and expressed from coconut kernels. It is stable when exposed to air. Coconut oil may be irritating to the skin and cause skin rashes. It is also considered comedogenic.

cocoyl sarcosine—its application in skin care products is not clear. It is formed from caffeine through decomposition with barium hydroxide.

collagen—very popular in skin care formulations for its great hydration potential and its ability to bind and retain many times its weight in water. This water-binding and retention ability makes collagen effective for use in skin moisturizers as a skin-protecting agent. An additional plus for formulators and consumers is that it will not leave a feeling of tackiness or dryness, especially when used as hydrolyzed or soluble collagen. As a film former, collagen aids in reducing natural moisture loss, thereby helping hydrate the skin. In skin care preparations it enhances the humectancy of a topical product, contributes sheen, builds viscosity, and leaves the skin smooth and soft. Collagen is not water soluble. It has been very popular in cosmetic formulations for 20 years. Collagen is considered a "commercially pure" protein found in animal connective tissue, and it is similar to the collagen produced by the body in the skin and bones. Also considered an anti-irritant, collagen does not cause allergic reactions when used on the skin. It is very stable, bland in odor, and light in color. This is one of the most effective and economical proteins available to cosmetic formulators.

collagen amino acids—has a higher moisture-binding capacity than collagen alone, thus improving the moisturizing efficiency of skin creams and lotions. Collagen amino acid is a mixture of amino acids resulting from the complete hydrolysis of collagen. Its moisture-binding capacity is due to the very large number of hydrophilic groups per unit weight. *See also* collagen.

collagen amino-polysiloxane hydrolyzate—*see* collagen.

collagen fiber—anti-irritant and hydrating. When used in particular sponge versions it can serve as a delivery system for active ingredients. Its total lack of solubility in water and other commonly used cosmetic ingredients have restricted its range of application.

collagen hydrolysates (AKA hydrolyzed animal protein; hydrolyzed collagen)—collagen processed to achieve a lower molecular weight than regular collagen, which facilitates its use in cosmetic formulations and improves the properties of regular collagen. This is one of the most common forms of collagen used in cosmetic formulations. *See also* collagen.

collagen (soluble)—demonstrates enhanced moisture uptake and therefore is more effective than collagen. This is a clear liquid form of collagen preferred for use in cosmetics because, when incorporated into a formulation, it will not separate as regular collagen would. When incorporated into detergents, soluble collagen significantly reduces the amount of amino acids extracted from the skin when washing with the detergents and water. Soluble collagen is perhaps the most widely used and recognized high-molecular-weight protein in skin care formulations. *See also* collagen.

colloidal oatmeal—an anti-itching skin protectant with soothing properties. Its lipid content gives it enhanced lubricity and emolliency. Colloidal oatmeal has consistently been recommended for use on infants, adults, and geriatrics in bath, lotion, and poultice preparations designed for topical application on damaged skin. The addition of colloidal oatmeal to bath water diminishes inflammation and irritation that frequently occur in eczema cases when bathing with soap alone. It is used in cleansing creams, soaps, and bath products. *See also* oat.

colloidal sulfur—*see* sulfur.

colostrum fraction P—when mixed with elastin in the same product, it leaves a colloidal film that mimics the natural elastin.

coltsfoot extract *(Tussilago farfara)*—has astringent and emollient properties. Coltsfoot extract contains a high concentration of mucilage, making it useful for soothing delicate and/or easily inflamed skin. The leaves are the primary plant part used, but the flower stems are also utilized.

comfrey extract *(Symphytum officinale)*—contains allantoin and is credited with healing, astringent, and emollient properties. It is used in cases of swelling and bruising, cuts, papules, and pustules. Comfrey extract was traditionally used topically for soothing and anti-itching treatments as well as for eczema and sunburns. The whole plant is considered excellent for soothing pain in any tender, inflamed, or suppurating part. Comfrey root's chief and most important constituent is mucilage, which it contains in great abundance. It also contains from 0.6–0.8% of allantoin and a bit of tannin. European rumors are that certain alkaloids found in comfrey are toxic. The roots and leaves are generally collected from wild plants.

copper—copper-based ingredients are used as coloring agents in cosmetics. Copper itself is nontoxic, but soluble copper salts, notably copper sulfite, are skin irritants. As an oligoelement, copper has a specific catalytic action in the keratinization process. In normal skin, this process is completed in 8–12 hours; more than three days may be required in cases of copper deficiency. Copper also plays an active role in melanin production as decreased pigmentation has been observed in cases of copper deficiency. Also, the enzymatic activity resulting from a presence of copper affects collagen formations.

copper aspartate—*see* copper.

copper gluconate—*see* copper.

copra oil—*see* coconut oil.

coriander oil *(Coriandrum sativum)*—used in the appropriate mixture and dosage, it can work with other natural oils and extracts as a preservative. It also serves as a deodorant. Coriander oil is produced from the distillation of the fruit (the so-called seeds), which contains about 1% of volatile oil—the active constituent. The fruit also contains malic acid. Coriander oil can cause allergic reactions.

corn cob meal—used in face and bath powders. Made from the ear of Indian corn.

corn germ oil—a skin softener derived from the germ of the seed of the corn plant.

corn meal—used as a thickening agent. It is a coarse corn flour prepared by milling the corn kernel. *See also* corn starch.

corn oil—used as a carrier. This vegetable oil has average emollient properties. Although not particularly prone to cause allergies, it is also not widely used in cosmetic formulations. It is considered somewhat comedogenic. Corn oil is obtained from the wet milling of corn.

corn seed extract—found in creams, lotions, and revitalizing ampoules. *See also* corn seed fraction.

corn seed fraction—credited with increasing skin metabolism. It is rich in amino acids, sugar, vitamin B, and phytates. Can be used in creams, lotions, and postsun preparations.

corn starch—used as a thickener in cosmetics and in face powders. Corn starch absorbs water and is soothing to the skin. It can cause allergic reactions such as inflamed eyes, stuffy nose, and perennial hey fever. A natural material obtained from corn kernels.

cornflower extract *(Centaurea cyanus)*—used in folklore as a tonic and stimulant with action similar to that of blessed thistle. A water distilled from cornflower petals was formerly in repute as a remedy for weak eyes. Cornflower extract has been used in Europe since ancient times to treat bites. Considered beneficial for normal skin and skin care products designed for use around the eyes. Healing properties, particularly in cases of bruises, are attributed to cornflower extract obtained from the plant leaves. Important constituents include gentiopricrin, erythrocentaurine, nicotinic acid compounds, essential oil, and oleanolic acid.

cornflower water—*see* cornflower extract.

cotton seed oil (hydrogenated)—a carrier. This oil is used in the manufacture of soaps, creams, and baby creams. Although it is known to cause allergies and be mildly irritating, it is widely used in cosmetics. Considered somewhat comedogenic. Expressed from various species of cotton.

crane's bill extract *(Geranium maculatum)*—credited with astringent and tonic properties. Constituents include gallic and tannic acid. The leaves and roots are the parts used.

cream—contains lecithin, sterols, and oils plus 18–40% butterfat. It is the yellowish part of cow's milk.

cresin—*see* ozokerite.

cryolidone—a PCA derivative. Cryolidone increases resistance to heat following UV radiation. It provides a cooling effect on the skin so is suggested as an ingredient for postsun and aftershave products.

cucumber extract *(Cucumis sativus)*—credited with moisture-binding, moisture-regulating, soothing, tightening, anti-itching, refreshing, and anti-inflammatory properties. It contains amino acids and organic acids that are claimed to strengthen the skin's acid mantle. This extract can be used in aftershave preparations, eye treatment products, and treatments for oily skin. It is also effective in emulsions as a tightening agent for tired, stressed skin and in sun preparations as a refresher. Important constituents include minerals, mucins, and amino acids. The fruit is the part used.

cyclomethicone—provides a silky, smooth feel to skin care products and is considered a noncomedogenic emollient. This is a form of silicone that can deliver active ingredients and also serve as a vehicle for delivering fragrance.

O-cymen 5-OL—a bactericide used in hand and body preparations. A phenol derivative.

cypress extract (*Cupressus* sp.)—an extract derived from the leaves and twigs of the cypress tree. *See also* cypress oil.

cypress oil—said to have antiseptic, astringent, healing, soothing, and antispasmodic properties. Cypress oil is also claimed useful in treating acne and in inhibiting oil gland secretion. It can also be used as a fragrance. This oil, which can range from clear to yellow to brown, is generally obtained from a distillation of cypress cones.

cysteine—an amino acid. Cysteine is a component of the skin's natural moisturizing factor and can help normalize oil gland secretion due to its sulfur content. It is also said to promote wound healing. Considered good for treating oily skin, cysteine is an essential amino acid obtained via fermentation.

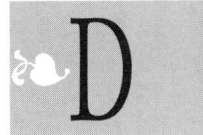

D&C colors—refer to color entry in chapter 4.

D-alpha-tocopherol—*see* vitamin E.

daisy extract *(Bellis perennis)*—said to be tonic. Daisy was a component in a popular fourteenth century wound ointment. This application continued through the centuries, using daisy alone or in combination with ox-eye daisy. The flowers and leaves are found to have a certain amount of oil and ammoniacal salts.

damiana leaves extract *(Turnera aphrodisiaca)*—the cosmetic properties of this spicy, aromatic extract are not clear, but they could be tonic and stimulant. The leaves, which are the part used, produce a greenish volatile oil that smells like chamomile and damianin, an amorphous bitter principle, resins, and tannin.

dandelion extract *(Taraxacum officinale)*—has tonic properties, refreshes the skin, and corrects pH balance. It apparently also aids in increasing the respiratory capacity of skin tissue. Dandelion extract is said to be beneficial for dry skin. The plant root, rather than the flower, is used in cosmetic preparations as the juice of the root is the more powerful part of the plant. The main constituents of dandelion root are taraxacin, a crystalline, bitter substance; and taraxacerin, an acrid resin. Other constituents include inulin, gluten gum, potash, citric acid, sterols, and vitamins B and C. Dandelion is used in many patented medicines.

DEA (AKA diethanolamine)—an organic alkali used in formulations to neutralize organic acids. Usually listed

D DEA cetyl phosphate

on ingredient labels preceding the compound that it is neutralizing. Oleth 3 phosphate, for example, is a powerful emulsifier, but when it is made it is very acidic so manufacturers use DEA to neutralize it. The organic alkali improves the nature of a formulation.

DEA cetyl phosphate—an emulsifying agent that gives a rich, velvety feel to a product. It can be used as a primary or secondary emulsifier, depending on the concentration. This is the diethanolamine salt of cetyl phosphate.

DEA oleth 3 phosphate—an emulsifier. This is the diethanolamine salt of a complex mixture of phosophoric acid esters and oleth-3.

DEA oleth 10 phosphate—an emulsifying agent used primarily in moisturizing preparations. This is the diethanolamine salt of a complex mixture of phosphoric acid esters and oleth-10.

DEA p-methoxycinnamate (octocrylene)—a chemical UV absorber that exhibits excellent UV absorption and has an approved usage level of 8–10%. Because of its water solubility it is not generally used in waterproof formulations.

decaglyceryl dipalmitate (AKA polyglyceryl-10 dipalmitate)—an emulsifier.

decyl alcohol—serves as an intermediate for surface-active agents. It is also an antifoam agent and a fixative in perfumes. Decyl alcohol occurs naturally in sweet orange and ambrette seed. It is also derived commercially from liquid paraffin.

decyl glucoside—a mild foaming cleansing agent.

decyl oleate—an emollient with good penetrating properties that facilitates product spreadability and provides a formulation with good feel on the skin. A component of the sebum of human skin, it is also produced synthetically and from olive oil.

decyl polyglucose—a nonionic surfactant with good foaming properties. It is extremely mild to the eyes and skin. It can be obtained from naturally derived raw materials from renewable sources, though this depends on the supplier.

dehydroacetic acid—a preservative with low sensitizing potential. This is a weak acid used as a fungi- and bacteria-destroying agent in cosmetics. The presence of organic matter decreases its effectiveness. It is not irritating or allergy causing when applied on the skin.

deoxyribonucleic acid—*see* DNA.

dermasomes—liposomal preparations containing cosmetic ingredients (usually actives) entrapped within lipid spheres. Dermasomes provide increased penetration and absorption, improved product efficiency at lower usage levels, and targeted and time-released delivery.

devil's claw *(Harpagophytum procumbens)*—said to have anti-inflammatory and moisture-binding capabilities. The plant's root contains mucilage.

dextrin (AKA British gum; starch gum)—absorbs moisture. This powder, produced from corn starch and modified via a bacterial process, may cause an allergic reaction. Used as a binder in cosmetic form.

dextrose—*see* glucose.

DHA—*see* dihydroxyacetone.

diatomaceous earth—in purified form, it is used for powders and as an abrasive agent in peeling formulations. If improperly formulated, it may be too abrasive as a peeling agent. Diatomaceus earth is a fine-grain, almost white powder consisting mostly of amorphous silicic acid that is obtained by crushing the silicic acid structures of monocellular sea algae.

diazolidinyl urea—an antiseptic and deodorizer. It is also a broad-spectrum preservative against bacteria and fungi. Generally, it is used in concentrations of 0.03–0.3%. It has been found that diazolidinyl urea is a stronger sensitizer than imidazolidinyl urea for people sensitive or allergic to formaldehyde.

dicetyl dilinoleate—a nonirritating emollient that provides slip; emollience; and a smooth, satiny feel to a cosmetic preparation. It leaves the skin feeling soft, supple, and without greasiness. It is claimed that dicetyl dilinoleate helps normalize the epidermal lipid structure and promotes the formation of soft, flexible, and healthy-looking skin. It may also act as a vehicle for the delivery of active topical substances. This ingredient can be effectively incorporated into creams, lotions, skin oils, and makeup bases that contain sunscreens. Dicetyl dilinoleate can be used instead of, or as a replacement for, partially hydrogenated animal and vegetable tallows, cocoa butter, and isopropyl lanolate. It is based on omega 6 linoleic acid, a naturally occurring vegetable derivative.

diethanolamine—*see* DEA.

diethanolamine p-methoxycinnamate—*see* DEA p-methoxycinnamate

diethyl lauramide—*see* lauramide DEA.

diethylene glycol monoethylene ether—*see* ethoxydiglycol.

digalloyl trioleate—an FDA-approved sunscreen chemical with an approved usage level of 2–5%. A chemical UVB absorber, digalloyl trioleate is no longer available as it apparently exhibits a poor UV absorption profile.

dihydroxyacetone (AKA DHA)—a self-tanning agent used in cosmetics designed to provide a tanned appearance without the need for sun exposure. It is also a UV protector and a color additive. As a self-tanning agent it reacts with amino acids found on the skin's epidermal layer. Its effect lasts only a few days as the color it provides fades with the natural shedding of the stained cells. Reportedly, it works best on slightly acidic skin. DHA, when combined with lawsone, becomes an FDA Category I (approved) UV protectant. In 1973 the FDA declared that DHA is safe and suitable for use in cosmetics or drugs that are applied to color the skin and has exempted it from color additive certification. Found naturally in the human body, and obtained by the action of certain bacteria on glycerol, thus far it has not been synthetically duplicated for use in formulations.

diisoarachidyl dilinoleate—a liquid wax emollient that provides good product spreadability. It may replace mineral oil in skin care preparations.

diisoarachidyl dodecanedioate—an emollient. This liquid wax provides a feel similar to heavy mineral oil but without the greasiness and oiliness associated with it. It may therefore be used as a partial or total replacement for mineral oil in formulations where improved tactile properties are sought. Diisoarachidyl dodecanedioate leaves a protective, though not completely occlusive, film on the skin. Its qualities suggest use in special cleansing preparations; rich, soft creams; and sunscreens. Considered a potentially excellent vehicle for the delivery of active topical substances. It is nonirritating in skin and eye tests.

diisocetyl dodecanedioate—an emollient that enhances refattening of the skin. This ingredient is made from low-irritation components.

diisopropyl adipate—a low-viscosity emollient. It increases a preparation's spreadability.

diisopropyl dimerate—a chemical modifier that lowers the irritation potential of other ingredients incorporated into a formulation.

diisostearyl dimer dilinoleate—an occlusive skin-conditioning agent primarily used in makeup and hand and body preparations.

diisostearyl malate—a film former and a secondary emollient used mostly in makeup or other formulations involving suspensions.

dimethicone—a form of silicone used to give products lubricity, slip, and good feel. It can also serve as a formulation defoamer and help reduce the effect that some creams have upon the skin with immediate application. It is also reported to protect the skin against moisture loss when it is used in larger quantities. It improves product flow and spreadability. In combination with other ingredients it becomes a very good waterproofing material for sunscreen emulsions and helps reduce the greasiness often seen in high-SPF preparations.

dimethicone copolyol—provides soft feel and helps reduce irritation caused by soap. Used to improve the skin feel of some sunscreen preparations. A modified form of dimethicone. *See also* dimethicone.

dimethicone copolyol isostearate—acts as a skin softener and gives a formulation high lubricity. *See also* dimethicone.

dimethiconol esters—fatty wax that liquifies when rubbed on the skin. *See also* dimethicone.

dimethiconol hydroxystearate—an oil-phase compound with nonocclusive hydrophobic film formation on skin. *See also* dimethicone.

dimethiconol stearate—a nonocclusive hydrophobic water-proofing base used in sunscreens and other skin care applications. *See also* dimethicone.

dimethyl isosorbide—a carrier. Its particular skin-penetrating ability opens the possibility of enhancing active substance efficacy in topical products. Its physical characteristics and solubility properties are superior to those of propylene glycol, glycerin, or ethyl alcohol.

dimethyl oxazolidine—a compound that improves the activity of a preservative present in a cosmetic formulation. It is nontoxic at approved cosmetic-use levels.

dimethyl siloxane—*see* dimethicone.

dimethylisosorbide—*see* dimethyl isosorbide.

dimethylsilanol hyaluronate—has very strong skin hydrating activity. It is said to provide regenerating, restructuring, and repairing action for tissue suppleness. Finds application in antiaging products and those for skin maintenance such as night, sun, and protective creams.

dioctyl adipate—an emollient. It allows transepidermal respiration through occlusive-type films. Has a very low irritancy level.

dioctyl malate—a light film former and emollient used in skin care formulations.

dioctyl maleate—a film former and emollient derived from maleic acid.

dioctylcyclohexane—an emollient used as a squalene substitute.

dioctyl sodium sulfosuccinate—a mild surfactant used as a cleansing agent.

dioxybenzone (AKA benzophenone-8)—an FDA-approved sunscreen chemical with an approved usage level of 3%. Its use in sunscreen formulations is being replaced by other chemicals, with statistics indicating a decline in use by manufacturers since 1986.

dipotassium phosphate—used as a buffering agent to control the degree of acidity in solutions.

dipropylene glycol monomethyl ether (AKA PEG 2 methyl ether)—used as a formula stabilizer and to improve skin penetration in topically applied acne preparations containing erythromycin.

disodium EDTA—a preservative used in concentrations of 0.1–0.5%.

disodium laureth sulfosuccinate—a very mild surfactant, appropriate for baby and child care products. It reduces the irritation properties of high-foaming surfactants when used in the same product formulation.

disodium mono-oleamido MIPA sulfosuccinanate—*see* dioctyl sodium sulfosuccinate.

disodium phosphate—considered a moisturizer. This inorganic salt absorbs moisture from the air that is then supposed to be released to the skin. In dry climatic conditions, however, it may draw moisture from the skin and release it to the air, aggravating dryness. Without water, disodium phosphate may cause slight irritation.

DL-alpha-tocopherol—*see* vitamin E.

DMDM hydantoin—a popular preservative with moderate sensitizing potential. It is used worldwide and is one of the fastest growing cosmetic preservatives, with an excellent safety record for use in leave-on and wash-off cosmetic preparations.

DNA (freeze-dried) (pure biological) (pure vegetal) (AKA deoxyribonucleic acid)—a surface film-forming protein with moisturizing action. It is claimed to be a more effective moisturizer than glycerin or collagen. DNA's large macromolecules do not enable it to penetrate the skin. In addition, its affinity with the corneum layer keeps it anchored to the skin's surface where it serves to protect and retain skin moisture. It is usually used in a potassium salt form obtained from fish sperm.

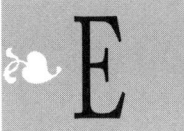

ECM—*see* extra cellular matrix.

EDTA—a preservative. *See also* ethylendiamine tetraacetic acid.

echinacea *(Echinacea angustifolia)*—described as having antiseptic and antibacterial properties helpful in the treatment of skin lesions and in shortening healing time. It also has anti-itching and soothing properties when used in skin care products. The main constituents of both the oil and the resin derived from the wood or bark of the plant are inulin, inuloid, sucrose, sulose, betaine, 2 phytosterols and fatty acids, oleic, cerotic, linolic, and palmatic.

egg lecithin—recommended for sensitive skin. *See also* egg protein; egg yolk extract.

egg oil—recommended for sensitive skins. It is extracted from the egg yolk using vegetable oil, thereby obtaining egg oil. *See also* egg protein; egg yolk extract.

egg protein—creates a film on the face, thereby acting as a moisture-retention agent, and allows the skin to build up a supply of water. This moisturization process tightens and softens the skin only temporarily as the skin cannot utilize the protein contained in an egg. Egg protein is used primarily in facial masks. It may cause skin rashes and other disorders in those with an allergy to eggs.

egg yolk extract—a protein with emulsifying capabilities used in products for sensitive skin. It contains lecithin sterols and vitamin A. This is an extract of egg yolk. It provides a temporary tightening effect on the skin. *See also* egg protein.

egg yolk powder—used in many cosmetics including face masks, creams, and bath preparations. It provides a temporary tightening effect on the skin. *See also* egg yolk extract.

Egyptian rose extract—*see* rose extract.

elastin—a surface protective agent used in cosmetics to alleviate the effects of dry skin, enhance flexibility, improve feel, increase and improve the tension of the skin, and influence formation of tropocollagen fibers when used with soluble collagen. Preparations containing elastin and peptides derived from it are reported to promote wound healing. Reportedly, in such systems, elastin can absorb lipids from the skin and, when applied to scars, increase the structural glycoproteins and elastin available in the scar tissue. Elastin is an elastic structural protein found in the dermis together with collagen and is difficult to obtain in pure form. Collagen and elastin are similar, though elastin has a different amino acid composition and is found in lower concentrations. Its molecular size is also much smaller than collagen's, and as a result there is a tendency to believe that it penetrates the surface epidermal layers thereby improving overall skin appearance, softness, and suppleness. Elastin's main application is as a surface-protective agent, though it is also used in products for aging or mature skin.

elastin (hydrolyzed)—a modified form of elastin that is more convenient for use in cosmetic formulations than regular elastin, which is far too insoluble in cosmetic media. Applications in skin care products are the same as those described for elastin. *See also* elastin.

elastin hydrolysates—*see* elastin (hydrolyzed).

elastin polypeptides—an elastin-derived ingredient that can be used as an active ingredient carried by liposomes.

elder extract (*Sambucus* sp.)—an herb that is said to have astringent, antiseptic, and emollient properties. It is useful for problem or inflamed skin. The bark, leaves, flowers, and berries have all been used botanically, though use of the bark is now considered obsolete. Ointments made of elder leaves have been domestic remedies for bruises, swelling, and wounds. Elder leaves are also an ingredient in many cooling ointments. Manufacturers report that presently the flower is the preferred segment of the plant.

elder flower extract—mildly astringent and a gentle stimulant. It is principally used as a vehicle for eye and skin lotions. It is reported to be particularly beneficial in treatment of dry skin. In the nineteenth century, elder flower water was commonly used to clear the complexion of freckles and sunburn and keep the skin in good condition. The most important constituent of elder flower is a trace of semisolid volatile oil, present in very low percentage, which possesses the scent of the flower in a high degree. *See also* elder extract.

elecampane *(Inula helenium)* (AKA horseheal; scabwort)—in centuries past its herbal properties for external use were described as astringent and antiseptic. It was used for treating skin problems in people and animals. Its common name, scabwort, comes from belief that it cured sheep affected with the scab. It gets its other name, horseheal, from its reputed virtues in curing skin diseases of horses. Elecampe's therapeutic value is attributed to its abundant content of inulin. The extract used for therapeutic purposes is preferably obtained from the root of a two- to three-year-old plant. When the plant is older the root becomes too woody for extraction.

elm bark (*Ulmus* sp.)—credited with astringent, healing, and soothing properties that could benefit surface skin problems.

elm extract—described as a problem skin extract due to its healing and reputed cicatrizant properties. Extracts from elm leaves have been recommended by herbologists to wash wounds, bruises, and sore eyes.

embryo extract (AKA embryonic extract)—originally used in special masks and facial applications in spas and skin care salons where it was prepared from eggs that had been incubated for 10 to 14 days of their total 21-day incubation period. The immediate results were apparently a visible difference in the look of the skin. An adjusted version of the original mix was incorporated into cosmetic products designed for aging or mature skin. The use of embryo extract in skin care cosmetics is based on the theory that its particular hormone content can rejuvenate the skin. This is a controversial concept as some scientists deny its validity, and professionals in esthetics claim otherwise. It becomes even more controversial when referring to retail cosmetics. It may cause an allergic reaction in people allergic to eggs. There is another version of embryo extract based on an oil-soluble extract of fetal calves, to which similar rejuvenating properties are being attributed.

embryonic extract—*see* embryo extract.

emulsifying wax—an emulsifier and thickening agent used to give body to a formulation. Unlike some waxes (e.g., beeswax), this is not a true wax. It is a chemical mixture of emulsifiers and fatty alcohols that permits the formulation of stable creams.

emulsifying wax NF—this is the same as emulsifying wax and is considered a noncomedogenic raw material. NF is the abbreviation for a reference called National

Formulary. It denotes quality compliance with the pharmaceutical monogram.

English daisy extract—said to reduce swelling. *See also* daisy extract.

English oak extract—*see* oak; quercus extract.

enzymes—refer to enzyme entry in chapter 4.

epidermal lipid extract—an example of a vague ingredient description found on some product labels. Literally this would be an oil or fat extracted from the epidermis. It is not specific enough to allow one to determine if lipids that blend with those in the human skin or lipids extracted from animal epidermis are being used.

ergocalciferol—*see* vitamin D.

escin—a saponin occurring in the seed of the horse chestnut tree. *See also* horse chestnut extract.

esculin—used as a skin protectant in ointments and creams. This is a glucoside compound originally obtained from the leaves and bark of the horse chestnut tree. *See also* horse chestnut extract.

ethanol—*see* ethyl alcohol.

ethanol acetamide—*see* acetamide MEA.

ethoxydiglycol—a solvent for essential oils, fragrance materials, and terpene oils. It is used primarily in nail enamels and rarely in skin care products. However, ethoxydiglycol is nonirritating, nonpenetrating, and noncomedogenic when applied to the skin.

ethoxyethanol—*see* ethylene glycol monomethyl ether.

ethyl alcohol—commonly known as rubbing alcohol. Ethyl alcohol is ordinary alcohol—ethanol—and is used medicinally as a topical antiseptic, astringent, and antibacterial. At concentrations above 15% it is also a broad-spectrum preservative against bacteria and fungi and can add to the adequacy of other preservatives in a formulation. Cosmetic companies tend to use alcohol SD 40 in high-grade cosmetic manufacturing as they consider ethanol too strong and too drying for application on the skin. Obtained from grain distillation. It can also be synthetic. *See also* alcohol.

ethyl 4-[bis(hydroxypropyl)] aminobenzoate—an FDA-approved sunscreen chemical with an approved usage level of 1–5%.

ethyl arachidonate—an emollient with healing and smoothing properties. Reported for use in indoor tanning preparations. It is the ester of ethyl alcohol and arachidonic acid. A modified form of ethyl arachidonate can reduce the possibility of irritation that can result from using straight ethyl arachidonate.

ethyl cellulose—a binder, film former, and thickener. It is used in suntan gels, creams, and lotions. This is the ethyl ether of cellulose.

ethyl dihydroxypropyl PABA (AKA ethyl dihydroxypropyl p-aminobenzoate)—an FDA-approved sunscreen chemical for UVB absorption. It exhibits the widest range of UV spectrum absorption abilities among UVB absorbers. Its structure results in very limited solubility by commonly used cosmetic solvents, so it is not among the more frequently used chemicals in its class. Due to its limited popularity, it was withdrawn from the marketplace in the early 1990s and is no longer available.

ethyl dihydroxypropyl p-aminobenzoate—*see* ethyl dihydroxypropyl PABA.

ethyl ether—a solvent that may cause skin irritation. Although considered a noncomedogenic raw material, it is rarely used in cosmetics.

ethyl linoleate (AKA vitamin F)—an emollient and an essential fatty acid. *See also* vitamin F.

ethyl linolenate—an emollient reportedly used in indoor tanning preparations. It is not very popular as it may pose rancidity problems.

ethyl paraben—a preservative with minimal sensitizing potential. *See also* parabens.

ethylene acrylate copolymer—film former, binder, and viscosity-increasing agent. A synthetic polymer. *See also* acrylates.

ethylene glycol monomethyl ether (AKA ethoxyethanol)—considered a noncomedogenic raw material. It is used as a solvent in nail products and a stabilizer in cosmetic emulsions. It is able to penetrate the skin and may cause skin irritation.

ethylene glycol monostrearate (AKA glycol stearate)—a noncomedogenic raw material that provides a pearly look and consistency to clear preparations. *See also* glycol stearate.

ethylenediamine tetraacetic acid—*see* EDTA.

2-ethylhexyl 2-cyano-3, 3-diphenylacrylate (AKA octylcrylene; UV absorber 3)—one of 21 FDA-approved sunscreen chemicals. As a UVB absorber, it has an approved usage level of 7–10%. It is being studied by many companies as a very effective SPF booster and a waterproofing enhancer. It may become increasingly popular.

2-ethylhexyl 2-hydroxybenzoate—*see* octyl salicylate.

2-ethylhexyl isostearate—a chemical reactant used in cosmetic formulations to reduce the amount of antioxidants needed for that particular formulation. Also an emollient for high-quality skin care preparations. This is an isosteric acid derivative.

2-ethylhexyl methoxycinnamate—*see* octyl methoxycinnamate.

ethylhexyl p-methoxycinnamate—*see* octyl methoxycinnamate.

2-ethylhexyl p-methoxycinnamate—see octyl methoxycinnamate

ethylhexyl-p—*see* octyl palmitate.

ethylhexyl palmitate—*see* octyl palmitate.

2-ethylhexyl salicylate (AKA octyl salicylate)—one of 21 FDA-approved sunscreen chemicals for UVB absorption. It has an approved usage level of 3–5%. It is a good solubilizer for benzophenone-3.

eucalyptol—considered an antiseptic. This is a monoterpene compound that provides the fragrance associated with the essential oil of eucalyptus. Eucalyptol is also used to fragrance cosmetic preparations. *See also* cajeput oil; eucalyptus oil.

eucalyptus extract *(Eucalytpus globulus)*—possibly a mild astringent with antiseptic properties. It may also act as an insect repellant. *See also* eucalyptus oil.

eucalyptus oil—described as having antiseptic, disinfectant, and blood-circulation-activating properties. It is also used as a fragrance. Native to Australia, it was regarded as a general cure-all by the Aborigines and later by the European settlers. It has a long tradition of use in medicine and is considered one of the most powerful and versatile herbal remedies. It is said that eucalyptus oil's antiseptic properties and disinfectant action increase as the oil ages, and ozone is formed in it when exposed to air. The most important constituent of the oil is eucalyptol. The essential oil is obtained from eucalyptus leaves. Eucalyptus oil may cause allergic reactions.

Eucerin—a trade name for a cosmetic preparation base.

evening primrose oil *(Oenothera biennis)*—has therapeutic botanical properties described as astringent and helpful for skin irritations. It contains a high amount of gamma linoleic acid, which is one of the essential fatty acids vital for the maintenance of normal functioning of the epithelial barrier membrane. Evening primrose oil improves the skin's ability to develop normal barrier functions.

everlasting oil *(Gnaphalium polycephalum)*—reported to decrease UVB-induced erythema on sunburned skin. If applied prior to sun exposure, it prevents the development of UVB-induced erythema. The photoprotective activities of this oil are largely due to the action of flavonoids.

extra cellular matrix (AKA ECM)—one of the new generation of skin care ingredients developed primarily for use on wrinkled, mature skin. ECM is described as a mixture of bioactive substances including collagen, glycosaminoglycans, heparan sulfate, dermatan sulfate, chondroitin sulfate, and the glycoproteins laminin and fibronectin. It has the ability to stimulate the cells to actually help repair the skin. In general, it is believed to improve cellular function.

eyebright extract *(Euphrasia officinalis)*—an herb credited with astringent, anti-inflammatory, and tonic properties. As indicated by its name, it has traditionally been used in eye care preparations to decrease and counteract eye area inflammation and potential irritations. Some manufacturer's claim that when combined with horsetail and lady's mantle it works to counter skin wrinkling around the eye area. Important constituents of eyebright extract include tannin, mineral salts, and iridic glycosides. The extract is prepared from the plant after it has been cut just above the root.

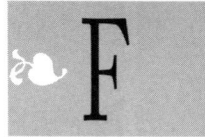

FD&C colors—refer to color entry in chapter 4.

fango—*see* mud.

fango mud—a redundancy, as *fango* means mud in Italian.

farnesol—described as a substance of high biological potential, capable of acting in the skin as a true bioactivator. Farnesol is said to help smooth wrinkles; normalize sebum secretion; and increase the skin's elasticity, tissue tension, and moisture-binding capacity. It is able to penetrate the epidermis. A biological precursor and a fatty alcohol, farnesol is one component of vitamin K. In humans it is found in the skin and is involved in sterol biosynthesis. It is widely present in vegetables and found in many essential oils (e.g., acacia, lilac, lily of the valley, rose, orange blossom, oakmoss, and sandalwood).

farnesyl acetate—a variety of beneficial effects on the skin's metabolic process have been noted with the use of compounds consisting of a mixture of farnesyl acetate, farnesol and panthenyl triacetate.

fennel extract *(Foeniculum vulgare)*—described as a cleanser and detoxifier indicated for use by oily skin types. The principal constituents of fennel oil are anethol and fenchone, plus d-pinene, phellandrine, anisic acid, and anisic aldehyde. Anethol, also a main constituent of anise oil, may produce hives, scaling, and blisters when applied to the skin. The therapeutic properties of fennel oil are most probably due to fenchone, and so only the varieties of fennel that contain a good proportion of fenchone are suitable for therapeutic use. Fennel oil is obtained from distillation of seeds.

fenugreek extract *(Trigonella foenum-graecum)*—considered an emollient, anti-inflammatory, and healing ingredient. It was traditionally used in treatments for irritated skin. The seeds of this annual herb have been used through the ages and were held in high regard among the Egyptians, Greeks, and Romans for medicinal and culinary purposes.

ferric ferrocyanide—a blue color with no known toxicity.

feverfew extract *(Chrysanthemum parthenium)*—used for its esters and borneol as a counterirritant. It is claimed to relieve the pain and swelling caused by insect bites. Feverfew is a perennial, herbaceous plant.

fibronectin—as a cosmetic ingredient it is described as a surface-protective agent with a moisturizing and protective effect. Fibronectin's function in the skin is to strengthen the attachments between collagen and elastin fibers, fibroblasts and other cells in the dermis, and other connective tissues. Its presence may also be important to cell growth. Research suggests fibronectin plays a significant role in maintaining a healthy basal layer. There is also some evidence that fibronectin may act as a cell regenerator by reversing abnormal cell formation and growth. Fibronectin is a glycoprotein and an important component of the skin's basal lamina. Produced by many types of cells, it is present in the skin primarily in the basal membranes. It constitutes 1–3% of the total cellular protein of fibroblasts. Fibronectin is manufactured from animal blood.

fibronectin (hydrolyzed)—a humectant and moisturizing agent for skin creams and lotions. *See also* fibronectin.

field poppy extract—therapeutic properties are described as pain and spasm soothing.

figwort extract *(Scrophularia nodosa)*—traditionally used in cases of superficial burns, including sunburns, cutaneous eruptions, swelling, and inflammations. There are a number of varieties of figwort, including common, yellow, balm-leaved, water, and knotted, all appearing to have similar properties. The extract is obtained from the plant's leaves.

fir needle—*see* pine needle extract.

firmogen—provides an astringent, strengthening, and tightening effect. Its use in cosmetic formulations results in smoother skin feel. Firmogen is a biological substance blending polysaccharides with hydrolyzed enzymatic proteins.

fish collagenic protein—a transparent, uncolored gel used in moisturizers.

fish glycerides—a fish oil used primarily in soaps.

five leaf grass—*see* cinquefoil extract.

flavonoids—antioxidants. *See also* bioflavonoids.

flavonastases—an enzyme. *See also* enzyme.

flowers extract—probably used as a fragrance. Such a listing is an all-encompassing statement that does not allow one to identify the type of flowers used and therefore prohibits one from determining any therapeutic value.

fluid oil—a play on words describing the physical state of the oil rather than the type of oil used. This does not allow one to identify the value or function of the oil in the cosmetic preparation.

folic acid—an emollient. Folic acid is a member of the vitamin B complex.

fragrance—refer to fragrance entry in chapter 4.

frankincense *(Boswellia thurifera)*—described as an anti-inflammatory agent and a mild antiseptic that brings relief to dry and sensitive skins and helps heal all types of wounds. Its astringent properties are said to help balance oily or overactive skin. This is one of the oldest essential oils in use and dates back to ancient Egypt.

fructose—a naturally occurring sugar in fruits and honey. It has moisture-binding and skin-softening properties.

fruit oil extract—a blend used in perfumery.

fucus—*see* seaweed extract.

fucus algae *(Fucus vesiculosus)* (AKA fucus seaweed)—a succulent giant kelp with some preservative and fragrance value. Its essential oil exhibits antimicrobial activity as it contains compounds similar to traditional preservatives.

fucus seaweed—*see* fucus algae.

fumitory herb extract *(Fumaria officinalis)*—has been credited with curative properties due to its purifying powers. The notes of European physicians of old attribute bleaching and skin-clearing properties to this extract. The leaves yield a juice credited with medicinal properties due to the presence of fumaric and malic acids. This is a small annual plant considered a common weed.

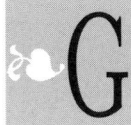

gallic acid—a potential bleaching agent. Scientists are finding that gallic acid may serve as a skin lightening agent by inhibiting the action of the tyrosinase and peroxidase enzymes. Some studies are indicating that it is more effective than hydroquinone when combined with the proper ingredients.

gamma linoleic acid—*see* linoleic acid.

garlic extract *(Allium sativum)*—many effects and healing powers have been attributed to garlic, which has long been recognized as an antiseptic and bactericide. In World War I it was used to control the suppuration of wounds. It is sometimes externally applied in ointments and lotions to reduce hard swellings and for treating problem skin (e.g., acne). The active properties of garlic depend on a pungent, volatile, essential oil that is obtained by distillation with water. This oil is a sulfide of the radical allyl present in the onion family, and it is rich in sulfur, but contains no oxygen. The common garlic is included in the same group of plants as the onion.

garlic oil—considered a healing oil with bacteriostatic and bactericidal action. It is incorporated into skin care formulations for skin healing and to aid in clearing problems such as eczema and acne. *See also* garlic extract.

garlic sage—*see* germander extract.

gelatin—used as a natural sealant against moisture loss and as a formulation thickener. The films produced by gelatin are tacky when moist and hard and brittle when dry. This is a product obtained by the partial hydrolysis of mature collagen derived from the skin, connective tissue, and bones of animals. It does not have the water-binding ability of soluble collagen.

gellan gum—used as a gelling agent, thickener, and stabilizer in cosmetic preparations.

genistein—may control excess sebum secretion by inhibiting oil gland activity and is therefore applicable in sebum-reducing preparations.

gentian extract (*Gentiana* sp.)—credited with cooling, antiseptic, and anti-inflammatory properties. All known gentian species are remarkable for their intensely bitter properties. Hence, they are considered valuable tonic medicines. The root is the principal part used for medicinal and cosmetic purposes. Dried gentian root contains gentiin, gentiamarin, and bitter glucosides, together with gentianic acid (gentisin) and gentiopicrin.

geranium oil (*Pelargonium* sp.)—botanical properties are described as refreshing, anti-irritant, mildly tonic, and astringent. Although good for all skin types, it is of particular benefit to oily and acne skins and those with inflammatory tendencies. The cell regenerating activities claimed for geranium would make it also useful for aged skin. In addition, this oil is widely used in perfumery and cosmetics. Although there are many varieties of geranium, including wild geranium and English geranium, all belonging to the same botanical family, their uses may be somewhat different. Geranium oil is obtained by steam distillation from the entire plant.

geranium burbon oil—*see* geranium oil.

Germall II—the trade name for imidazolidinyl urea. A preservative. *See also* imidazolidinyl urea.

germander extract *(Teucrium scorodonia)* (AKA garlic sage; wood sage)—credited with astringent and tonic properties. Noted as useful for skin problems and wounds. The whole herb is used for manufacturing the extract.

GHPT—*see* guar hydroxypropyltrimonium chloride.

ginkgo biloba extract (AKA ginkgo extract)—used in folkloric medicine as a blood vessel dilator with the ability to increase blood flow and to function as a stimulator of tissue oxygen consumption. It is also said to have a positive protective effect on vascular walls, thus diminishing couperose condition, as well as antioxidant properties, thereby protecting the skin against free radicals. These properties make it an effective ingredient in "antiaging" cosmetic formulations. Its important constituents include catechin, tannin, quercetin, and luteolin.

ginkgo extract—*see* ginkgo biloba extract.

ginseng extract *(Panax* sp.)—a number of therapeutic benefits have been associated with ginseng. Folkloric remedies cite use for boils, bruises, sores, and swellings. Ginseng is considered tonic and is believed to be nourishing due to its vitamin and hormone content. It seems to aid in diminishing wrinkles and help dry skin. It is also said to aid in increasing skin elasticity, perhaps due to a stimulation of sterol and protein production. Other claims include skin rejuvenating, oxygenating, and stimulating. This root's active components are called ginsenosides and are said to be responsible for the revitalization and reactivation of epidermal cells. Important constituents include saponins, mucin, vitamin B, and ginsenoside. There are various types of ginseng, with *Panax ginseng* being the most frequently used. The extract comes from the root. Ginseng has been associated with many allergic skin reactions.

ginseng root extract—a redundancy as the therapeutic portion of the plant used is the root. *See also* ginseng extract.

glucans—studies indicate an ability to stimulate immune system activity, thereby helping the body fight a variety of infectious diseases caused by bacterial, fungal, viral, and parasitic organisms. Glucans also seem to have antitumor activity. *See also* polyglucan.

glucoronic acid—a chelating agent, pH adjuster, and humectant that gives a smooth feel to the skin.

glucose—has moisture-binding properties and provides the skin with a soothing effect. It is a sugar that is generally obtained by the hydrolysis of starch.

glucose glutamate—a humectant for hand creams and lotions and a skin conditioner and moisturizer that enhances lather in surfactant systems. Glucose glutamate is the ester of glucose and glutamic acid and is considered a noncomedogenic, nonirritating raw material.

Glucoviton—a trade name referring to a mixture of glucoronic acid and Hydroviton.

glutamic acid—a moisture binder and an antioxidant. Glutamic acid is an amino acid manufactured via fermentation generally from a vegetable protein.

glutaral (AKA glutardialdehyde)—a broad-spectrum preservative that can cause skin irritation. This is an amino acid occurring in green sugar beets.

glutardialdehyde—*see* glutaral.

glutathione—believed to enhance the skin's cellular metabolism and oxygen utilization. It has been found to protect the fibroblast against toxic action caused by oxidation. A plant and animal tissue component.

glutathione peroxidase—helps control inflammation. Its most frequent application is in shaving preparations.

glycereth-26—*see* glycerin.

glycerin (AKA glycerol; propanetriol)—a humectant used in moisturizers due to its water-binding capabilities that allow it to draw and absorb water from the air. Glycerin helps the skin retain moisture. Like other low-molecular-weight glycols, glycerin was thought to be an ideal moisturizer. However, if used under aggressive climatic conditions such as excessive wind, sun, and dryness, it has been found to absorb moisture from the skin rather than from the air where the relative humidity is low, thus contributing to a dry skin feeling. Glycerin also improves the spreading qualities of creams and lotions. It is a clear, syrupy liquid made by chemically combining water and fat that is usually derived from vegetable oil. While glycerin has not been shown to cause allergies, in concentrated solutions it may be comedogenic and irritating to the mucous membranes.

glycerin monostearate—*see* glyceryl monostearate.

glycerine—*see* glycerin.

glycerol—a glycerin alcohol. *See also* glycerin.

glycerol stearate lipophilic—*see* glycerin.

glyceryl—a glycerin ester. *See also* glycerin.

glyceryl aminobenzoate (AKA glyceryl PABA)—in actuality it should be listed as glyceryl p-aminobenzoate. This is an FDA-approved sunscreen chemical for UVB absorption with an approved usage level of 2–3%. It is, however, too water soluble to be effectively used in waterproof formulations, and its use raises safety concerns about the presence of benzocane.

glyceryl arachidonate—an emulsifier and emollient with moisturizing properties. It is reportedly used in suntan gels, creams, and lotions.

glyceryl caprylate—a coemulsifier, solubilizer, and surfactant that promotes absorption and has bacteriostatic action in cosmetic formulations.

glyceryl isostearate—*see* glyceryl mono-isostearate.

glyceryl laurate—a coemulsifer for oil-in-water emulsions. It is also a superfattening agent that promotes absorption and has a bacteriostatic effect.

glyceryl linoleate—an emollient with moisturizing capabilities. It is synthetically produced from naturally derived ingredients.

glyceryl mono-isostearate (AKA glyceryl isostearate)—an isostearic acid often incorporated into cosmetic formulations as an emollient.

glyceryl monostearate (AKA glycerin monostearate; glyceryl stearate)—widely used in cosmetics. It functions as an emulsifying and solubilizing ingredient, dispersing agent, emollient, formula stabilizer, and surface-active agent for a wide variety of products. Employed in baby creams, face masks, foundation, and hand lotions. It is often derived from hydrogenated soybean oil. Glyceryl monostearate has little or no toxicity. *See also* glyceryl stearate.

glyceryl oleate—an emollient and stabilizer derived from olive oil. A water-in-oil emulsifier that allows for softer emulsions than glyceryl stearate.

glyceryl PABA—*see* glyceryl aminobenzoate.

glyceryl ricinoleate—an emollient and an emulsifier used in the preparation of creams and lotions.

glyceryl stearate—an emulsifier that assists in forming neutral, stable emulsions. It is also a solvent, humectant, and consistency regulator in water-in-oil and oil-in-water formulations. It may also be used as a skin lubricant and imparts a pleasant skin feel. Glyceryl stearate is a mixture of mono-, di-, and tri- glycerides of palmitic and stearic acids and is made from glycerin and stearic fatty acids. Derived for cosmetic use from palm kernel or soy oil, it is also found in the human body. It is very mild with a low skin-irritation profile. A slight risk of irritation exists if products have poor-quality glyceryl stearate.

glyceryl stearate lipophilic—*see* glyceryl stearate.

glyceryl stearate SE—self-emulsifying glyceryl stearate. Provides a stable, uniform oil-in-water emulsion. *See also* glyceryl stearate.

glyceryl tri-isostearate (AKA triisostearin)—an emollient and emulsifier.

glyceryl trioctanoate—an emollient with skin-softening abilities.

glycine—an amino acid used as a texturizer in cosmetic formulations. It makes up approximately 30% of the collagen molecule.

glycoceramides—it is suggested that the topical application of glycoceramides helps replenish intercorneal lipids and regulate the skin's ability to bind and retain moisture. In addition, it improves the ability of hydrophilic and hydrophobic materials to traverse the corneum layer (the movement of water into the skin and removal of by-products of cell metabolism from the skin). This ensures the intercelluar regulatory balance and enhances and restores the barrier function. Glycoceramides can be incorporated into emulsions.

glycocoll—*see* glycine.

glycogen—a skin-conditioning agent. It is a high-molecular-weight polymer distributed through the cell protoplasm.

glycol propylene—*see* propylene glycol.

glycol stearate—can be utilized as a detergent, emulsifier, surfactant, thickener, stabilizer, and emollient in cosmetic formulations. It converts clear cleansers to ones that are pearly.

glycolic acid (AKA hydroxyacetic acid)—research indicates that glycolic acid reduces corneocyte cohesion and corneum layer thickening where excess dead skin cell buildup can be associated with many common skin problems. Glycolic acid acts by dissolving the intercellular cement responsible for abnormal keratinization. It also appears to improve skin hydration by enhanced moisture uptake as well as increased binding of water to the stratum corneum. This leads to a sloughing of dead skin cells that has demonstrated effectiveness in helping clear the pores of acne-prone skin; smoothing the fine lines in older, photo-aged skin; and diminishing the signs of actinic keratosis, commonly referred to as age or liver spots. It provides relief to thick, dry skin. Glycolic acid is found in sugar cane. It is the simplest alpha hydroxyacid (AHA) and is the one scientists and formulators believe has penetration potential because of its small molecular weight. It is mildly irritating to the skin and the mucous membranes. *See also* alpha hydroxyacid.

glycolipids—emulsifiers and moisturizers. *See also* glycoprotein (soluble).

glycoprotein—a skin-conditioning agent derived from carbohydrates and protein. *See also* glycoprotein (soluble).

glycoprotein (soluble)—a group of proteins found in the intercellular layers, the best known of which is fibronectin. It is found in the cellular matrix of the dermis and plays a role in cell migration during wound healing. The mechanism by which it might provide cosmetic benefits has not yet been clearly established. *See also* fibronectin.

glycosaminoglycans (AKA mucopolysaccharides)—one of the newest cosmetic ingredients. Glycosaminoglycans are used in cosmetics for their ability to increase depth hydration and, with this, the elasticity and pliability of the skin. Glycosaminoglycans are credited with moisturizing and firming properties. They reportedly leave the skin smooth and with a pleasant, velvety softness and evenness and minimize wrinkle appearance. They are easily accepted by the skin due to their high charge and affinity. The mechanism by which this ingredient might provide cosmetic benefits is not clear. Although not exactly the same component as mucopolysaccharides, this is the scientifically preferred name for a group of materials that include chitin, chondroitin sulfates, heparin, and hyaluronic acid. In the form of proteoglycans they are derived from cartilaginous fish. They can also be derived from umbilical cord, avian combs, and calf connective tissues.

glycoside/C-12-16—a mixture of synthetic fatty alcohols with 12 to 16 carbons in the alkyl chain.

glycosphingolipids—a more recent development in ingredient technology for skin care product formulation. It is believed that when used in facial creams, glycosphingolipids replenish the lipids lost from the skin and renew the skin's barrier function and moisture-binding capacity. When incorporated into aftershave preparations, they also seem to help soothe nicks and cuts. Laboratory studies prove that glycosphingolipids can reduce transepidermal water loss when applied to the skin, even at 5% in a typical oil-in-water emulsion. Although references are made to its performance, being such a new ingredient the mechanism by which its benefits might be provided are not entirely clear. Glycosphingolipids, comprised of lipids and sugars, are a class of molecules embedded in the membranes of cells throughout the body where they act to regulate the interaction of healthy cells with their environment.

glycyrrhetic acid—*see* 18 beta-glycerrhentinic acid.

glycyrrhetinic acid—anti-irritant, antiallergenic, anti-inflammatory, and smoothing properties are attributed to this ingredient, which is also a carrier. It is the organic compound derived from glycyrrhizic acid or shredded licorice roots.

glycyrrhizic acid—a hydrolyzed glycyrrhizin. It is credited with anti-inflammatory and antiallergenic properties. Studies comparing glycyrrhizin with hydrocortisone found glycyrrhizin to be somewhat milder but longer lasting in effectiveness. Once the application of hydrocortisone is suspended the symptoms return. This does not appear to be the case with glycyrrhizin. It does not have side effects and is chemically stable so it can be safely used on a continuing basis. *See also* licorice extract.

goldenrod extract (*Solidago* sp.)—considered to have antiseptic action and recommended for use in acne products to discourage the spread of infection through skin pustules. The extract is made from various species of *Solidago virgaurea*, principally from the plant leaves.

goldenseal extract *(Hydrastis canadensis)*—reported to be effective in the treatment of eczema, itching, and wounds. Native Americans valued the root for its general ulceration-healing properties. The extract is made from the plant's rhizomes. Goldenseal extract's main constituents are the alkaloids berberine, hydrastine, and canadine. The rhizome is said to be much more alkaloid rich than the root.

gotu kola extract *(Centella asiatica)* (AKA hydrocotyl or *Hydrocotyl asiatica*)—traditionally used for couperose condition. It was also used for soothing and anti-itching treatment in dermatological disorders. In addition, gotu kola is considered healing. It is helpful against sunburns and other superficial, though not extensive, burns.

grape—used in extract form, it is described as tonic. Grape's main constituent is a high proportion of berberin, with oxycanthin also present. Grapes also contain vitamin C, chlorophyll, and enzymes. The value of these components to the skin is based on the method of extract processing and cosmetic manufacturing.

grapefruit extract *(Citrus paradisi)*—reported as having antiseptic properties. It is indicated as beneficial for oily skin. Fresh grapefuit juice contains vitamin C and is very acidic. As such, in high concentrations it is too caustic to use on the skin and face. There should be no problem, however, at normal use levels. The extract obtained from the juice is preferred over that from the rind as there is practically no vitamin C available in the rind. Furthermore, unless properly obtained and processed, fertilizers and insecticide residues on the rind may provoke blemishes and allergic reactions in sensitive people. As vitamin C is considered an unstable component, grapefruit extract's value in cosmetics depends on the method of extraction and the product's formulation.

grapefruit oil—used as a fragrance and also as an active component with anti-irritant properties. Grapefruit oil is believed to help control the liquid process and as such is indicated for work with the lymphatic system.

grapefruit seed extract—said to have antibacterial properties. This is the extract from the seeds of the grapefruit. *See also* grapefruit extract.

grapeseed extract—considered a counterirritant with soothing and antibacterial properties. *See also* grape.

grapeseed oil—has moisturizing and nourishing properties due to its high linoleic acid content. Grapeseed oil is the fixed oil obtained by pressing grapeseeds.

green apple extract—*see* apple extract.

green clay—*see* clay.

green tea extract—contains catechins that are potent antioxidants. May also have bacteriostatic action. *See also* tea extract.

guaiac extract *(Guaiacum officinale)*—credited with antiseptic and stimulating properties. Resin with therapeutic properties is extracted from the hard wood of the guaiac tree.

guanine—color. It is mixed in water and used primarily in nail polish to achieve a pearlized effect. It has been greatly replaced by either synthetic pearl or aluminum and bronze particles. Guanine is obtained by scraping the scales of certain fish (e.g., alewives and herring).

guar gum—has a coating action on the skin that allows for moisture retention. Often used as a thickener and emulsifier in cosmetic formulations, guar gum is a polysaccharide found in the seeds of a specific plant. It is the nutrient material required by the developing plant embryo during germination. When the endosperm, once separated from the hull and embryo, is ground to a powder form it is marketed as guar gum.

guar hydroxypropyltrimonium chloride (AKA GHPT)—an anti-irritant and anti-inflammatory that is also used as a thickening, conditioning, and antistatic agent. It helps maintain a product's smoothing action. Some manufacturers cite it as also having skin-softening capabilities. It imparts excellent skin conditioning in creams or lotions that otherwise may not be used on the face. It adds lubricity to a product when in contact with the skin. There is some evidence that it can enhance a formulation's viscosity and stability. A derivative of guar gum.

gum acacia—*see* acacia.

gum Arabic—*see* acacia.

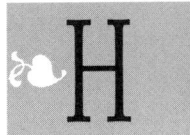

hamamelis (AKA winterbloom; witch hazel)—*see* witch hazel.

hamamelis (dry) extract—claimed botanical properties include anti-free radical, UVB absorber, healing, soothing, and anti-itching activity. *See also* witch hazel.

hawthorn extract *(Crataegus oxyacantha)*—sources cite it as having active ingredients with valuable therapeutic properties such as antispasmodic, vasodilator, and sedative. Obtained from the berries, flowers, and/or leaves of hawthorn.

hayflower extract—reported to activate the circulatory system, have analgesic properties, and provide a tightening effect on the skin. Historically, hayflower extract was used in Europe to stimulate the circulation and for rheumatic complaints. Its many active constituents include essential oils, vitamin D, amino acids, carotinoids, caffeic acid, 4-methoxycinnamic acid, and tannin. This extract has a faintly sweet fragrance. Hayflower is not a specific plant but rather a mixture that is formed by the leftover blossoms and leaves in a hay loft.

hazel nut extract—an herb said to have astringent properties.

hazel nut oil—a carrier oil also described as having some nourishing properties. As a carrier, it imparts excellent lubricity, pale color, and low odor. This oil is used in products designed for dry skin. Obtained from the nuts of various species of the hazelnut tree.

hectorite—one of the principal constituents of bentonite clay. Used as a thickener and suspending agent in water-based systems in oil-in-water emulsions.

helichrysum oil—*see* everlasting oil.

henna extract *(Lawsonia insermis)*—primarily a colorant that provides a reddish brown hue to products. It is also a conditioner. Henna's properties are described as antiseptic and astringent. Important constituents include mucins, phytosterols, and naptho quinones. Generally, the extract is obtained from the leaves.

heptane—a solvent and viscosity-decreasing agent.

hexadecanol—*see* cetyl alcohol.

N-hexadecyl-n, n, n-trimethylammonium-*trans*-retinoate—has some effect in inhibiting the *P. acnes* bacteria associated with acne formation.

hexamidine—a preservative.

hexyl laurate—a mild emollient and a vehicle for lipid-soluble active ingredients. Nonirritating and practically odorless. It gives a product excellent spreadability and feel on skin. *See also* lauric acid.

hexyl nicotinate—penetrates rapidly and dilates blood vessels, thereby temporarily activating blood circulation. This increased blood flow results in an enhanced supply of oxygen, nutrients, and moisture to the skin cells, along with a faster elimination of wastes via the metabolic process.

hexylene glycol—could be considered a solubilizer. *See also* polyethylene glycol.

hibiscus *(Hibiscus* sp.)—its properties are described as refreshing. It provides a tightening effect without stripping the skin of its natural oils. Hibiscus is a botanical recommended for oily skin due to its high degree of astringency and its tonifying properties. There are about 200 varieties of this plant whose extract is obtained from the flowers, which contain a number of vegetable acids and pigments.

histidine—a skin-conditioning amino acid. *See also* amino acid.

holy thistle—*see* blessed thistle extract.

homomenthyl salicylate—a chemical UVB absorber included in the FDA's Category I Sunscreen Chemical list. Its approved usage level is 4–15% by the FDA and 10% by the European Economic Community's Cosmetic Directive.

homosalate—*see* homomenthyl salicylate.

honey—although honey has no special properties for the skin, masks containing honey create a watertight film on the face and permit the skin to rehydrate itself. Given this, it can be said that honey has softening and moisturizing characteristics. Its use in cosmetics is centuries old and can be traced back at least to ancient Egypt and Cleopatra. Honey is composed of a variety of sugars, wax, and other substances, including citric, malic, formic, and lactic acids; beta carotene; enzymes; amino acids; and vitamins. It is a saccharic secretion produced enzymatically from flower nectar that is gathered and stored in honeycombs by honey bees. Honey may cause an allergic reaction in people allergic to pollen.

honey extract—an extract obtained from honey. *See also* honey.

honeysuckle extract *(Lonicera fragrantissima)*—botanical uses for external application include cutaneous tonic, protection against sunburns, and overall skin clearing. A dozen or more of the 100 different species of honeysuckle have botanical applications. Apparently, the leaves have more effect than the flowers.

honeysuckle oil—a biological additive with properties similar to those of honeysuckle extract.

hops extract *(Humulus lupulus)*—general effects attributed to hops include sedative, antiphlogistic and promotion of wound healing. Hops are also considered to have preservative value. Their use is claimed effective in acne products. Important constituents include humulone, lupulone, amino acids, chlorogenic acid, rutin, quercatin, flavonoids, and a lupamaric acid. The oil and the bitter principle combine to make hops more useful than chamomile or gentian. Hops extract is made from the cones of the hops vine and can cause allergic reactions.

horse chestnut extract *(Aesculus hippocastanum)*—benefits attributed to this botanical include antiphlogistic, spasmolytic, and circulation promotion. It apparently also has the ability to help reduce the permeability of capillaries. This would make it useful in cases of fragile or broken capillaries. Its tannic acid content provides horse chestnut extract with toning and astringent properties. Horse chestnut is recommended for use in products designed to stimulate circulation and normalize circulatory disorders. Suggested for use in creams for improving circulation and in bath salts for the stimulation of the whole organism. Some suppliers cite a recommended dosage of 2–5% for use in creams and emulsions and others cite 1–10% for bath and hair products. Detected constituents include starch, sugar, protein, tannis, oil, vitamins, phytosterol, and an easculus saponine content. The extract is usually obtained from the seed (fruit).

horseheal—*see* elecampane.

horseradish extract *(Armoracia lapathifolia)*—traditionally used against sunburns, superficial and other nonextensive burns, and to give the skin clarity and freshness. Its antiseptic and skin-clearing properties are linked to its ascorbic acid content. The extract is made primarily from the plant's roots.

horsetail extract *(Equisetum arvense)* (AKA shave grass)—general botanical properties include stimulating, healing, and softening. Horsetail is also described as able to increase the skin's defense mechanism, regulate the skin due to the plant's rich mineral content, and even strengthen connective tissue due to the presence of silicic acid. Some product manufacturers state that when mixed with lady's mantle and eyebright extracts it works to prevent and counteract wrinkles in the eye area. This is an extract of the sterile caules of *Equisetum arvense*, a fern plant whose sprouts have high silicic acid content as well as flavone glycosides and saponine. Amino acids such as citrulline, valine, asparaginic acid, lucine, and serine have also been detected as constituents of this extract. The recommended usage level is 1–10% of a formulation's total composition.

hortensis extract—*see* savory.

hyaluronic acid—a glycosaminoglycan component. Hyaluronic acid occurs naturally in the dermis. Its water-absorption abilities and large molecular structure allow the epidermis to achieve greater suppleness, proper plasticity, and turgor. Hyaluronic acid is a natural moisturizer with excellent water-binding capabilities. In a solution of 2% hyaluronic acid and 98% water, the hyaluronic acid holds the water so tightly that it appears to create a gel. However, it is a true liquid in that it can be diluted and will exhibit a liquid's normal viscous flow properties. When applied to the skin, hyaluronic acid forms a viscoelastic film in a manner similar to the way it holds water in the intercellular matrix of dermal connective tissues. This performance and behavior suggests that hyaluronic acid makes an ideal moisturizer base, allowing for the delivery of other agents to the skin. Manufacturers claim that the use of hyaluronic acid in cosmetics results in the need for much lower levels of lubricants and emollients in a formulation, thereby providing an essentially greaseless product. Furthermore, its ability to retain water gives immediate smoothness to rough skin surfaces and significantly improves skin appearance. Initially, hyaluronic acid was obtained from cock's combs and other animal sources. Because the extraction and purification procedures are very complex and expensive, scientists are now developing ways to produce hyaluronic acid from a nonanimal source.

hyaluronidase—its moisturizing properties are credited with improving skin elasticity, reducing skin dryness, and increasing the skin's moisture content by 33%. It is reported to have a greater moisturizing effect when used in conjunction with hydrolyzed protein than when used alone. In the skin, hyaluronidase is an important component of glycosaminoglycan.

Hydrocotyl asiatica—*see* gotu kola extract.

hydrocotyl extract—*see* gotu kola extract.

hydrogen peroxide—a bleaching and oxidizing agent, detergent, and antiseptic. Generally recognized as a safe preservative, germ killer, and skin bleacher in cosmetics. If used undiluted, it can cause burns of the skin and mucous membranes.

hydrogenated tallow octyl dimonium chloride—a conditioner used in clear or emulsion systems. It provides a soft feel and is lubricating in skin care products.

hydrolyzed animal protein—refers to processed collagen and other animal proteins that allow for better product performance in cosmetic formulations. It has been established that hydrolyzed collagen and elastin penetrate inside the skin and bind with 10 to 15 layers of the corneum layer to increase their moisture content. The primary function of these proteins is to form a glossy film on the skin. However, depending on the degree of hydrolysis, properties change from mostly film forming for moisture-loss reduction to individual amino acids that can penetrate the top layers of the corneum layer. The process of hydrolysis, commonly produced via enzyme hydrolysis, breaks the bonds of the larger molecules making them into smaller and smaller ones until finally one gets the amino acids themselves. Manufacturers hydrolyze the proteins in controlled environments to obtain the desired chain length appropriate for the properties of their formulations. The name listed as such does not indicate any specific level of hydrolysis. *See also* animal protein; collagen; collagen hydrolysates.

hydrolyzed collagen—*see* collagen hydrolysates.

hydrolyzed corn protein—forms a film on the skin's surface. It is used to reduce loss of the skin's natural moisture. *See also* hydrolyzed vegetable protein.

hydrolyzed elastin—forms a film on the skin's surface. A processed form of elastin that facilitates its use in skin care formulations. *See also* elastin (hydrolyzed).

hydrolyzed fibronectin—a humectant and moisturizing agent for skin creams and lotions. It is a processed form of fibronectin that facilitates its use in skin care formulations. *See also* fibronectin.

hydrolyzed glycosaminoglycans—has hygroscopic properties and a small molecular structure that favors penetration into the outer epidermal layers. This ingredient contains low molecular weight oligosaccharides and can be found in hydrating cosmetics. Recommended for stressed and aging skin. *See also* glycosaminoglycans.

hydrolyzed golden pea protein—forms a film on the skin's surface. This is a water-soluble liquid protein derivative and a vegetable protein of interest because of its high soluble tyrosine content. Tyrosine is considered to play an important role in stimulating cell growth and is an integral component of tyrosinase, which is responsible for the formation of melanin. Considered by some as the best replacement for hydrolyzed animal protein. *See also* hydrolyzed vegetable protein.

hydrolyzed keratin—a processed form of keratin that facilitates its use in skin care formulations. *See also* hydrolyzed animal protein; keratin.

hydrolyzed milk protein—forms a film on the skin's surface that allows the skin to retain moisture. This is a processed form of milk protein that facilitates and improves performance in skin care formulations. *See also* milk protein.

hydrolyzed mucopolysaccharides—helps skin hydration due to its strong water-binding properties that help decrease transepidermal water loss. This is a mixture of polysaccharides derived from the hydrolysis of animal connective tissue. *See also* mucopolysaccharides.

hydrolyzed oat protein—an anti-itching skin protectant with a soothing effect on sensitive skin. Its lipid content provides improved lubricating and emollient properties. This is a very smooth vegetable protein, derived by acid, enzyme, or other method of hydrolysis. *See also* hydrolyzed vegetable protein; oat; oat protein.

hydrolyzed potato protein—a vegetable protein that serves as a moisturizing agent. Reported to have a unique amino acid profile, with reasonable levels of the sulfur-containing amino acids cystine and methionine. This is the hydrolysate of potato protein derived by acid, enzyme, or other method of hydrolysis. *See also* hydrolyzed vegetable protein.

hydrolyzed rice protein—a vegetable protein that serves as a good moisturizing agent. This is the hydrolysate of rice protein derived by acid, enzyme, or other method of hydrolysis. *See also* hydrolyzed vegetable protein.

hydrolyzed serum proteins—a film-former and skin-conditioning substance that reduces transepidermal water loss and has anti-irritant properties It is also nourishing to the cells. *See also* hydrolyzed animal protein; serum protein.

hydrolyzed vegetable protein—forms a protein-lipid film on the skin, giving products a moisture-retention capacity. These proteins are obtained from wheat, soybean, corn, peas, or other vegetable sources. They are made by the hydrolysate of vegetable protein derived by acid, enzyme, or other method of hydrolysis. Some vegetable proteins have at least theoretically a composition that can make them appealing as a replacement for animal protein. Animal protein can be extracted almost as pure protein, but vegetable proteins have different levels of carbohydrates. In general vegetable proteins exhibit a different behavior from animal proteins, which affects the chemical reaction, additive requirements, and cosmetic product stability.

hydrolyzed wheat protein—offers conditioning, moisturizing and film-forming properties. It is an effective moisturizer in skin care products, where it helps retain moisture in the skin. It is used in almost all applications where hydrolyzed animal protein would traditionally be used. It is produced by an enzymatic hydrolysis of wheat gluten. *See also* hydrolyzed vegetable protein.

hydrolyzed wheat protein (AMP isostearoyl)—a skin-conditioning ingredient. This is a neutralized, alcohol-soluble wheat protein/fatty acid condensate. It can be found in skin tonics. *See also* hydrolyzed vegetable protein; hydrolyzed wheat protein.

hydrolyzed wheat protein polysiloxane copolymer—upon drying, it forms a protective conditioning film on the skin that reduces water loss. This is a wheat protein attached to silicone, which enhances the effects of protein and silicone on the skin. *See also* hydrolyzed wheat protein.

hydrolyzed whole wheat protein—a modified form of wheat protein to facilitate its performance and incorporation in skin care formulations. *See also* hydrolyzed wheat protein.

hydrolyzed yeast—the hydrolysate of yeast derived by acid, enzyme, or other method of hydrolysis. *See also* protein; yeast.

hydrotriticum wheat amino acids—an ingredient with good moisture-retention properties. It is reportedly able to penetrate the corneum layers and moisturize from within.

hydroquinone—a pigment-lightening agent used in bleaching creams. The FDA allows a maximum of 2% concentration in a cosmetic formulation. Although it occurs naturally, the synthetic version is the one commonly used in cosmetics. Hydroquinone combines with oxygen very rapidly and becomes brown when exposed to air. Application to the skin may cause allergic reaction.

Hydroviton—a trade name for a natural moisturizer derived from rose water, plant sugars, and plant-sourced amino acids. It contains glycerin, sodium lactate, TEA-lactate, serine, lactic acid, urea, sorbitol, lauryl diethylenediaminoglycine, lauryl aminopropylglycine, and allantoin.

2-hydroxy-p-methoxycinnamate—*see* cinoxate.

5-hydroxy-2-hydroxymethyl-γ-pyridone—a skin-lightening agent apparently 32 times more effective than kojic acid.

hydroxyacetic acid—*see* glycolic acid.

hydroxyacetone—*see* dihydroxyacetone.

hydroxyethyl cellulose—suggested as a thickener, protective colloid, binder, stabilizer, and suspending agent. It is obtained from wood pulp or chemical cotton by treatment with an alkali. *See also* ethyl cellulose.

hydroxylated lanolin—a modified form of lanolin. It increases the tackiness, stickiness, and emulsifying capacity of lanolin. A good suspending agent. It is obtained by the controlled hydroxylation of lanolin. *See also* lanolin.

6 hydroxy-5-methoxyindole—used as a skin pigmenter (i.e., to create a tanned look as with dihydroxyacetone). Said to yield the pigmentation level that would be obtained from natural tanning.

hydroxyoctacosanyl hydroxystearate—a consistency-regulating agent for water-in-oil emulsions used to improve the body of an emulsion. Used in creams, liquid makeup, and lipsticks. This is a synthetic beeswax substitute.

hydroxyproline—a skin-conditioning amino acid. It is a component of collagen.

hydroxypropyl methylcellulose—improves foaming properties, lubricity, and formula stabilization. May enable formulators to reduce the active surfactant concentrations without loss of the desirable lathering properties and result in a milder product. Mild to the skin and eyes. *See also* cellulose gum.

hydroxypropyltrimonium hydrolyzed wheat protein—enhances skin moisturization. This is considered an upgraded version of hydrolyzed wheat protein, particularly with respect to moisturizing properties. It is also a mildness agent for surfactants.

hydroxyproylated y-cyclodextrin — helps prevent skin roughness.

8-hydroxy stilbenes—a skin-lightening compound. It inhibits melanin formation by inhibiting tyrosinase activity. Does not cause skin irritation.

6 hydroxy-2,5,7,8-tetramethylchromatin-2-carboxyic acid—a free radical inhibitor. Studies indicate it penetrates the skin more effectively than vitamin E. Can be used in moisturizing lotions.

hypericum extract *(Hypericum perforatum)*—*see* St. John's wort extract.

hyssop oil *(Hyssopus officinalis)*—properties attributed to this oil include healing, tonic, and stimulating. It can also be used as a fragrance. Hyssop oil is indicated for dermatitis, eczema, and wounds because of its cicatrizant properties. An infusion of the leaves is reportedly used externally for the relief of muscular rheumatism, bruises, and discolored contusions. The oil is obtained from the distillation of the whole plant in flower.

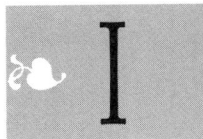

Iceland moss extract *(Cetraria islandica)*—used in cosmetics for its tonic properties. Despite its name, this plant is not a moss but rather a lichen containing about 70% lichen starch plus fumaric acid, oxalic acid, cetrarin, and licheno-stearic acid.

imidazolidinyl urea—one of the most commonly used antibacteria preservatives. The increase of its popularity among cosmetic formulators between 1977 and 1990 is credited to its low sensitizing potential. Today, it is the third most frequently used preservative in the United States. Generally, imidazolidinyl urea is not used alone but as a copreservative with parabens for broad-spectrum activity. Although it may yield low levels of formaldehyde when subjected to destructive methods, such as exposure to high temperatures, under normal use conditions there is no detection of free formaldehyde release. Of all the formaldehyde-releasing preservatives, imidazolidinyl urea is the one least likely to cause skin sensitization and allergic reactions. *See also* urea.

imidurea—an abbreviated annotation for imidazolidinyl urea. *See also* imidazolidinyl urea.

immunoglobulins—an ingredient being tested for use in anti-acne cosmetic preparations given its potential ability to decrease the *P. acnes* count by about half after one week of use. Obtained from cow's milk.

Indian chestnut extract—*see* chestnut extract.

inositol—used in emollients and belongs to the vitamin B family. While found naturally in plant and animal tissue, for commercial use it is isolated from corn.

iodopropynyl butylcarbamate—a preservative with broad fungicidal activity for use in skin care products. It is recommended for use in difficult formulation systems.

iris extract (*Iris* sp.)—The juice of fresh iris root has been employed as a cosmetic and freckle remover. There are many varieties of iris, many of which have a considerable reputation for their medicinal virtues. The *Iris versicolor* variety produces an official drug in the *U.S. Pharmacopoeia*.

Irish moss—*see* carrageen extract.

iron oxide—an inorganic compound frequently used to add color to cosmetics. It may have some slight sunscreening ability. Iron oxide can vary in color from red to brown, black to orange or yellow depending on the purity and amount of water added.

iron oxide (black)—*see* iron oxide.

iron oxide (red)—*see* iron oxide.

iron oxide (yellow)—*see* iron oxide.

isoarachidyl neopentanoate—an emollient with SPF-enhancing ability. It is generally used in sunscreen preparations. Considered noncomedogenic.

isobutyl paraben—a preservative.

isocream—an emollient. This is a mixture of mineral oil, lanolin, petrolatum, and lanolin alcohol.

isocreme—*see* isocream.

isodecyl citrate—a chemical compound used in formulations to inhibit the peroxidation of skin lipids. Often used in such items as antiaging creams and lotions, sunscreen preparations, and other skin care cosmetics.

isodecyl isononanoate—an emollient with a very low irritancy level that gives the skin a light, dry feel. Considered noncomedogenic.

isodecyl oleate—an emollient and moisturizer with wetting and pigment-binding properties.

isodecyl paraben—a preservative.

isododecane—a solvent.

isoflavones—a new ingredient with an apparent ability to inhibit sebaceous gland activity and reduce oil formation and flow. These properties would make it an excellent ingredient for oily and acne skin. It is currently being tested for use in skin care preparations.

isoparaffin—a solvent and diluent now rarely used in cosmetics.

isoprene glycol—a possible substitute for propylene glycol. It has good humectant properties, rubs nicely on the skin, and does not leave a greasy feeling. Isoprene glycol is also compatible with a variety of other organic chemicals commonly used by cosmetic formulators. Tests show good tolerance with respect to toxicity and irritation.

isopropanol—*see* isopropyl alcohol.

isopropyl alcohol—a carrier, antibacterial, and solvent for skin care lotions. Isopropyl alcohol is made from propylene, a petroleum derivative.

isopropyl hydroxycetyl ether—an emollient and skin-conditioning ingredient.

isopropyl isostearate—an emollient that leaves the skin surface with a smooth and supple finish. Isopropyl isostearate is a derivative of isostearic acid. *See also* stearic acid.

isopropyl lanolate—a skin softener that aids in the proper spreading of a product. It can also assist in extract penetration. A lanolin derivative. *See also* lanolin.

isopropyl myristate—an emollient, moisturizer, and skin softener that also assists in product penetration. A natural source is the myristic acid fraction of coconut oil. Myristic oil is also found in nutmeg. Although isopropyl myristate is generally considered comedogenic, some ingredient manufacturers clearly specify noncomedogenicity on their data sheets.

isopropyl palmitate—an emollient and moisturizer that can be derived from coconut oil. Similar to isopropyl myristate, it is produced from the combination of palmitic acid (coconut or palm oil) and isopropylic alcohol. Enzymes are able to metabolize this ingredient and studies do not show allergic reactions or toxicity. Some sources indicate a comedogenicity potential.

isopropyl stearate—an emollient and moisturizer. It leaves the skin with a smooth and supple finish. *See also* stearic acid.

isosorbide monolaurate—lends greaseless emollience to creams, lotions, and stick formulations. Permits formulation of nongreasy, very emollient lotions.

isostearamidopropyl PG dimonium chloride—an emulsifier/conditioner that leaves the skin with a soft, smooth feeling. Is not subject to oxidation or rancidity and has a very mild toxicological profile.

isostearic acid—an emollient that forms a lipid film on the skin permeable to water vapor, oxygen, and carbon dioxide. Isostearic acid is recommended for use in moisturizing cosmetics. This fatty acid is similar to waxes secreted by birds for feather maintenance.

isostearyl alcohol—an emollient and viscosity builder derived from isostearic acid. It gives the skin a silky feel after product application.

isostearyl isostearate—an emollient resembling jojoba oil. It leaves an almost imperceptible afterfeel. Some sources cite it as comedogenic with a slight irritancy potential. This is a derivative of isostearic acid.

isostearyl neopentanoate—an emollient, binder, and skin-conditioning agent with a moisturizing and softening effect. It has minimal allergenicity potential.

isostearyl stearoyl stearate—an occlusive skin-conditioning agent able to increase the viscosity of a formulation.

isothiazolin 3 one—a mixture that acts as a preservative against bacteria, fungi, and yeast. It is nontoxic at use levels of 0.02–0.1%, though it is severely irritating at concentrations of 1.5%.

isotretinoin—a retinoid derivative with improved bioavailability and percutaneous absorption for acne treatment products.

ivy extract *(Hedera helix)*—said to have a slimming and anti-cellulite effect due to its ability to prevent water accumulation in the skin tissue. Ivy extract is considered antibactericidal and soothing, particularly in burn cases. Apparently, ivy also has detergent, antiparasitic, decongestant, and analgesic properties. It is currently being studied for its vasoconstrictive and antiexudative properties given its vitamin P content and ability to reduce capillarian wall permeability. This extract seems to improve massage tolerance of sensitive skin areas as well. It lowers tissue sensitivity, activates circulation, and helps reduce local inflammation. Ivy extract contains saponines, foaming emulsion stabilizers, and surface active agents that assist in ingredient penetration and the emulsification of fats. Ivy is effective as a circulation stimulant in shower gels and in bath salts for "orange peeled" and bloated skin. In herbal medicine, a decoction of ivy leaves was traditionally used to treat various skin eruptions and skin ulcers. Fresh ivy leaves were used to dress wounds and pus-exuding sores. Ivy leaves themselves can cause skin irritation and dermatitis.

J

jasmine extract *(Jasminum officinale)*—a fragrance. Some ill-defined and unclear medicinal properties have been attributed to the root extract of several varieties of the 150 jasmine species. These properties include the difficult-to-prove benefit of stimulating the fibroblast with an increase in epidermal cell turnover. Jasmine may cause allergic reactions such as swelling. *See also* jasmine oil.

jasmine oil—fragrance. Credited with moisturizing, soothing, and healing properties. Given these, it is indicated for dry and sensitive skins and also for skin with dermatitis condition. In truth, there is no essential oil of jasmine. The essence is extracted through a very time-consuming and costly process, making jasmine oil one of the most expensive oils available. This can lead to the use of adulterated versions. Its sweet odor is so delicate and unique that until recently artificial or synthetic production was believed impossible. Today, synthetic otto of jasmine exists, however a portion of the natural oil must be added to the synthetic mixture to make the product satisfactory. The oil is extracted by a process known as enfleurage. The freshly gathered flowers are sprinkled over oiled glass trays and the flowers are renewed every morning while the plant is in bloom. Finally the pomade is scraped off the glass, melted at as low a temperature as possible, and then strained. When olive oil is used, flower petals are placed on coarse cotton cloths previously saturated with the olive oil. The cloths are squeezed under a press, yielding what is termed *huile antique au jasmin*. The oil of jasmine is later separated from the olive oil. Jasmine oil may cause allergic reactions, such as swelling, which may last several days.

jojoba oil *(Simmondsis chinensis)*—a moisturizer and emollient. Jojoba oil was traditionally held in high regard by Native Americans of the Sonora Desert for its cosmetic properties. Mystical properties have been attributed to it for its apparent ability to heal the skin. Jojoba oil reduces transepidermal water loss without completely blocking the transportation of water vapor and gases, providing the skin with suppleness and softness. In addition, it gives cosmetic products excellent spreadability and lubricity. Studies indicate a rapid penetration ability via absorption by the pores and hair follicles. From these areas it seems to diffuse into the corneal layer and act with intercellular lipids to further reduce water loss. Ingredient manufacturers claim that the chemical composition, functionality, blending ability, appearance, and feel of synthetically produced jojoba oil is the same as the natural oil. Jojoba oil is not a primary skin irritant and does not promote sensitization. Jojoba oil is a naturally occurring ester. Although it is generally considered noncomedogenic, laboratory studies indicate slight to moderate comedogenicity depending on the potency of the oil.

jojoba esters—an emollient and skin-conditioning agent made from jojoba oil and jojoba wax. *See also* jojoba oil.

jojoba wax—employed as a natural scrub bead in scrub gels, scrub soaps, and exfoliating products. Jojoba wax is hydrogenated jojoba oil. *See also* jojoba oil.

jonquil—*see* narcissus flower extract.

juniper extract *(Juniperus communis)*—a fragrance considered a mild skin stimulant. In botanical lore it is believed to help stimulate fibroblast growth, often resulting in increased epidermal cell turnover. *See also* juniper oil.

juniper oil—antiseptic, astringent, cleansing, and toning if used properly. Also credited with good penetration capabilities. Juniper oil is considered helpful in treating acne and good for use with oily skin. It is also indicated for dermatitis and eczema. Obtained from the distillation of the plant's small branches, juniper oil can be irritating in improper amounts.

juniper berry oil—effective for treating acne. Juniper berry oil has the same properties as those of juniper oil, but it is extracted from the plant's berry rather than its small branches. A distillation of the berries yields the best quality oil.

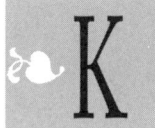

kaolin (AKA China clay)—a mixture of various aluminum silicates. It is often used in powders and masks. This white, soft powder has good coverage and absorption abilities for both water and oil, making it an appropriate absorber of the oil and sweat secreted by the skin. It adheres well to the skin's surface yet is easily removed with normal cleansing procedures. Kaolin is considered a noncomedogenic raw material.

kaolin China clay—*see* kaolin.

karite (unsaponifiable)—one of a group of vegetable oils with a small molecular structure, capable of penetrating and possibly becoming involved in the biochemical process of the dermis. It is considered a biological precursor. Karite contains steroidal and triterpenic structures. It is believed that the unsaponifiable fraction of karite can stimulate the dermal fibroblast to synthesize collagen, elastin, proteoglycans, and glycoproteins.

karite butter—*see* shea butter.

kelp—a marine product derived from the giant Pacific kelp. *See also* seaweed extract.

keratin—a surface protective agent with film-forming and moisturizing action. Keratin is often used in cosmetics for its moisture retention and protective effect. *See also* protein.

keratin amino acids—a mixture of amino acids obtained from the complete hydrolysis of keratin. *See also* amino acids; keratin.

khus-khus—*see* vetiver oil.

kiwi powder—used in scrubs for its abrasive properties. Obtained from ground kiwi seeds.

kojic acid—a skin-lightening agent of widespread use in Japan. Studies are finding it to be a tyrosinase inhibitor, though not as effective as licorice extract. When combined with allantoin and other proper ingredients in sunscreen preparations, the mixture can inhibit UV-caused erythema and accelerate wound healing.

kojic acid dipalmitate—preparations containing kojic acid dipalmitate are said to inhibit UV-induced erythema. *See also* kojic acid.

kojic acid monostearate—a kojic acid derivative said to inhibit tyrosinase and thus the formation of melanin. Kojic acid monostearate is used in skin-bleaching preparations. *See also* kojic acid.

kola extract *(Cola acuminata)*—largely known for its stimulating, astringent, and healing properties, research has also established anti-inflammatory and anti-irritant properties. These are achieved in part by blocking the penetration of specific chemical compounds. This extract may be used for dressing wounds. Kola extract is also somewhat effective for preventing viable epidermal penetration of certain substances. It has a high content of caffeine and other stimulants. The extract is obtained from the kola nut.

kukui nut oil *(Aleurites moluccana)* (AKA candlenut)—the kukui nut tree was used by early Hawaiians to soothe cuts and burns and to help protect the skin from damage due to sun and surf. Kukui nut oil is reported to have excellent penetration properties and to aid in soothing and moisturizing the skin and relieving chapped skin and irritations. This oil does not leave the skin with a greasy afterfeel. Kukui nut oil is apparently an excellent treatment for psoriasis and eczema and is also beneficial for acne and other common skin disorders. In addition, it is a sunscreen solubilizer that reduces the greasy feel often associated with sun products. Recent studies indicate possible natural sunscreen capabilities of its own, and when used with other sunscreens it may enhance a formulation's efficacy. Native to Hawaii, the nuts and kernels are roasted and then pressed for their clear oil, which has a high linoleic and linolenic acid content usually supplemented and stabilized with vitamins A, C, and E.

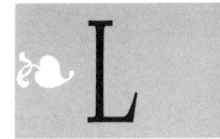

lactamide MEA—a surfactant that can also act as a thickener, foam booster, and stabilizer.

lactic acid (AKA sodium lactate)—a multipurpose ingredient used as a preservative, exfoliant, and moisturizer and to provide acidity to a formulation. In the body, lactic acid is found in the blood and muscle tissue as a product of the metabolism of glucose and glycogen. It is also a component of the skin's natural moisturizing factor. Lactic acid is an alpha hydroxyacid occurring in sour milk and other lesser-known sources such as beer, pickles, and other foods made through a process of bacterial fermentation. Lactic acid has better water intake than glycerin. Studies indicate an ability to increase the water-holding capacity of the corneum layer. They also show that the pliability of the corneum layer is closely related to the absorption of lactic acid (i.e., the greater the amount of absorbed lactic acid, the more pliable the corneum layer). Investigations report that continuous use of preparations formulated with lactic acid in concentrations ranging between 5 and 12% provide a mild to moderate improvement in fine wrinkling and softer, smoother skin. Lactic acid is caustic when applied to the skin in highly concentrated solutions.

lady's mantle extract *(Alchemilla vulgaris)* (AKA alchemilla)—said to have UV absorption ability for both the UVA and UVB spectrums. Other properties include anti-free radicals, healing, and anti-inflammatory. Its use is effective in acne treatment products. Herbalists of old considered lady's mantle extract one of the best wound herbs. This botanical was credited with drying wounds, reducing inflammation, and promoting quicker healing. Though the root was seldom used, an extract of fresh root was considered valuable to stop all bleedings. The active constituents of this perennial plant include tannins, rendering it effective against irritation, itching, and skin burns. Lady's mantle extract contains silicon/silicic acid, and it is reported that when combined with eyebright and horsetail, they all work synergistically to strengthen connective tissue.

laneth-10—an emulsifier that is particularly effective for emulsifying lanolin. It is the polyethylene glycol ether of lanolin alcohol.

laneth-10-acetate—an emulsifier. This is the acetylated ester of an ethoxylated ether of lanolin alcohol. *See also* laneth-10.

lanolide—a vegetable-derived substitute for lanolin. It is believed to be a good substitute because of its absence of pesticides, antiparasitic constituents, and heavy metals. These can be present in lanolin and have caused quite a few problems in the cosmetic industry.

lanolin—an emollient with moisturizing properties and an emulsifier with high water-absorption capabilities. Some consider lanolin a natural wax. Controversies surrounding this ingredient include a potential pesticide content and potential comodogenicity. There is a move among high-quality lanolin manufacturers to produce low pesticide lanolins and among high-quality cosmetic formulators and manufacturers to use the best form, in terms of purity, available. With respect to comodogenicity, this ascribed property is increasingly debated as some researchers believe it to be inaccurate, especially when lanolin is used in an emulsion. Lanolin has been found to form a network on the skin's surface rather than a film as is the case with petrolatum (Vaseline). Lanolin is a sheep's wool derivative formed by a fatlike viscous secretion of the sheep's sebaceous glands.

lanolin (hydrogenated) — a lanolin derivative. *See also* lanolin.

lanolin USP (modified)—an emollient and an emulsifier. This is a highly purified lanolin meeting USP monograph specifications that require analysis for trace contaminants. *See also* lanolin.

lanolin acetate—a lanolin derivative. *See also* lanolin.

lanolin alcohol—widely used as an emulsifier and emollient in water-in-oil systems. It absorbs a considerable amount of water that is then slowly released for moisturization purposes. Lanolin alcohol is a mixture of organic alcohols obtained from the hydrolysis of lanolin. It may cause skin sensitivity and allergic reactions.

lanolin oil—a lanolin derivative. This is the liquid fraction of lanolin obtained by physical means from whole lanolin. *See also* lanolin.

lanolin wax—a lanolin derivative. This is the semisolid fraction of lanolin obtained by physical means from whole lanolin. *See also* lanolin.

lanolin derivatives—a mixture of unspecified lanolin-derived products. *See also* lanolin.

lappa extract—*see* burdock extract.

lasilium—*see* sodium lacate methylsilanol.

lauramide DEA (AKA lauric acid diethanolamide)—a thickener, foam stabilizer, and viscosity builder in cosmetic formulations. It is added to liquid detergents and cleansers of the lauryl sulfate type to help stabilize the lather and improve foam formation.

laurel *(Laurus nobilis)* (AKA bay laurel)—when used in oil form, it is said to have antiseptic and astringent properties. This would make it effective for healing and skin problems. The oil is pressed from the berries and leaves.

laureth 2—a surfactant and emulsifying ingredient. It is the polyethylene glycol ether of lauryl alcohol. Increasing the number of moles (i.e., laureth 3, laureth 7, etc.) usually makes the product milder. *See also* lauryl alcohol.

laureth 3—a surfactant, detergent, and emulsifier used in cosmetic preparations. *See also* lauryl alcohol.

laureth 7—a wetting agent also used as an emulsifier, surfactant, detergent, and solubilizer for active substances. *See also* lauryl alcohol.

laureth 12—a surfactant, detergent, and emulsifier in cosmetic formulations. *See also* lauryl alcohol.

laureth 23—an emulsifier used with more frequency in oil-in-water than water-in-oil emulsions, though it is effective in both. It is also an emulsion stabilizer and can act as a surfactant. Laureth 23 may cause very minor irritation to skin and eyes. *See also* lauryl alcohol.

lauric acid (AKA *n*-dodecanoic acid)—due to its foaming properties, its derivatives are widely used as a base in the manufacture of soaps, detergents, and lauryl alcohol. Lauric acid is a common constituent of vegetable fats, especially coconut oil and laurel oil. It is a mild irritant but not a sensitizer, and some sources cite it as comedogenic.

lauric acid diethanolamide—*see* lauramide DEA.

lauroamphocarboxyglycinate—an organic cleansing agent that removes oil and dirt but can be slightly irritating to the skin.

lauroamphodiacetate—a mild cleansing agent.

lauroyl methionine lysinate—a free radical scavenger used in antiaging skin care cosmetics.

lauroyl lysine—an amino acid that also serves as a skin-conditioning agent. *See also* lysine.

lauryl alcohol—used in chemical formulations for a variety of purposes including as an emulsion stabilizer, a skin-conditioning emollient, and a viscosity-increasing agent.

lauryl aminopropylglycine—a skin-conditioning agent.

lauryl diethylenediaminoglycine—a skin-conditioning ingredient that appears to have greater application in hair formulations, where it is reported to work as an antistatic agent.

lauryl lactate—an emollient, detergent/emulsifier, and surfactant used in cosmetic formulations.

lauryl methyl gluceth-10 hydroxypropyl dimonium chloride—benefits include anti-irritancy, conditioning, humectancy, and moisturization.

laurylmethicone copolyol—an emulsifier that, when used in the proper concentration and with other emulsifiers, has excellent waterproof properties.

lauryl PCA—an emulsifier that has good affinity with skin lipids. It can increase a product's moisturizing action by decreasing transepidermal water loss. Lauryl PCA is a lipophile moisturizer with a delayed and remnant effect. Also used as a thickener or viscosity-control agent, it is derived from natural raw materials. This is the lauric ester of PCA.

lauryl sarcosine—a surfactant for cosmetic formulations.

lavender flower oil—the principal constituent of lavender is the volatile oil of which the dried flowers contain 1.5%–3%, while fresh flowers yield about 0.5%. This particular oil is pale yellow, yellowish green, or nearly colorless. Oil distilled from the earliest flowers is pale and contains a higher proportion of the more valuable esters. The oil distilled from the later flowers has a preponderance of the less valuable ester and is darker in color. Lavender oil owes its delicate perfume primarily to its esters. In the oil there are two esters that practically control the scent. Of these, the principal one is linalyl acetate and the second is linalyl butyrate. *See also* lavender oil.

lavender green oil—*see* lavender flower oil; lavender oil.

lavender oil *(Lavandula officinalis)*—a fragrance. Lavender oil is considered an all-purpose oil credited with many medicinal and folkloric properties. These include anti-allergenic, anti-inflammatory, antiseptic, antibacterial, antispasmodic, balancing, energizing, soothing, healing, tonic, and stimulating. In addition, it is said to help clean little wounds after washing and regulate skin functions. It may also have insect repellent properties. Lavender oil works well on all skin types and produces excellent results when used for oily skin as well as in the treatment of acne, burns (sunburns as well as other superficial and nonextensive types), dermatitis, eczema, and psoriasis. Its benefit to the dermis is immediate since it is easily and rapidly absorbed by the skin. Lavender oil is said to normalize any skin type and stimulate cellular growth and regeneration. When added to other oils, lavender can enhance and balance their effect. Lavender is also claimed to help relieve stress and as such is believed useful in treating skin problems caused or aggravated by stress. The known use of this oil extends at least to the Roman era when it was a popular additive to baths. From this practice and the Roman *lavare* meaning to wash, it derives its name. The oil's main component is linalool acetate, with other actives including geraniol, borneol, ocimene, and pinene. Lavender oil is distilled by using the flower tops and stalks. It is generally considered nontoxic, nonsensitizing, and nonirritating.

lawsone with dihydroxyacetone—one of the 21 FDA-approved sunscreen chemicals and listed as a Category I UVB absorber. Its approved usage level is 3%. Dihydroxyacetone (DHA) alone is used as a self-tanning agent in self-tanning products. DHA and lawsone together act as a sunscreen.

lecithin—a natural emollient, emulsifier, antioxidant, and spreading agent, lecithin is a hydrophilic ingredient that attracts water and acts as a moisturizer. Generally obtained for cosmetic products from eggs and soybeans, it is found in all living organisms.

lemon balm—*see* balm mint oil.

lemon bioflavonoids extract—obtained by extraction of oil rind. *See also* bioflavonoids; lemon extract.

lemon extract *(Citrus limonum)*—its botanical properties are described as antibactericidal, antiseptic, astringent, and toning. Lemon extract is suggested for treating sunburn, acne problems and oily skin. This extract contains citric acid and vitamins B and C. It can cause irritation and allergic reactions.

lemon oil—as one of the most versatile essential oils in aromatherapy it is considered a counterirritant, antiseptic, depurative, and lymphatic stimulant. The volatile oil is obtained from the fresh peel of *Citrus limon* (citrus lemon) that contains an essential oil and a bitter principle. Crystals of the glucoside hesperidin are deposited by the evaporation of the white, pulpy portion when boiled in water. Diluted acids decompose it into hesperidin and glucose. The oil is more fragrant and valuable if obtained by expression rather than distillation. Lemon oil can cause an allergic reaction.

lemon peel—*see* lemon oil.

lemongrass oil *(Cymbopogon citratus)*—considered astringent and tonic. It is widely used in the perfume and soap industries. Lemongrass oil is the volatile oil distilled from the leaves of the lemon grasses.

lettuce extract *(Lactuca virosa)*—said to have emollient properties in its fresh state, but after processing for use in cosmetics this property is unlikely to be retained. Herbologists attribute a sedative, narcotic property to lettuce extract. It is obtained from wild lettuce (not the garden and salad variety), a plant growing to a maximum height of 6 feet. The whole plant is rich in milky juice that flows freely from any cut made to it.

lichen extract—a preservative that can be used against certain types of bacteria, fungi, and yeast. It also contributes to the activity of other preservatives. Lichen extract is a water-free, natural, active agent extracted from alpine lichen. Nontoxic and nonirritating to skin.

licorice extract *(Glycyrrhiza glabra)*—considered an anti-irritant, studies indicate an ability to absorb UV rays in the A and B regions. Studies also conclude licorice extract has a depigmenting effect as well as an inhibitory effect on melanin synthesis due to its ability to act as a tyrosinase inhibitor. As a depigmenting agent, licorice extract is described as more effective than kojic acid and 75 times more effective than ascorbic acid. The chief constituent of licorice root is glycyrrhizin present in concentrations that range from 5 to 24%, depending on the variety of licorice used. A member of the bean family, licorice's pharmacological properties are found in the plant's roots and stem.

licorice root extract—*see* licorice extract.

lily extract—there are almost 100 different known varieties of lilies to which antiseptic and skin-clearing properties are generally ascribed. Herbalists have also ascribed demulcent (soothing) and astringent properties to the Madonna lily variety. The extract from the bulbs of this variety is said to be used primarily for its emollient, healing, soothing, and anti-inflammatory action. The extract from leaves and roots of the white pond lily variety has been described as astringent, healing, and anti-inflammatory.

lime blossom extract—a perfume ingredient. It is also an emollient with soothing and antiseptic properties. Lime blossom extract is a source of vitamin C. It can cause adverse reactions when the skin is exposed to sunlight.

lime oil *(Citrus acida, Citrus aurantifolia)*—has similar properties and uses as lemon oil. Lime oil is extracted from lime skin by cold pressure or distillation. *See also* lemon oil.

lime tree extract—the main extract from the lime tree is the one obtained from the blossoms. Some extract may also be obtained from leaves and sap. Lime tree is sometimes referred to as linden. *See also* linden extract.

linden extract *(Tilia* sp.)—the bark extract can be used to help problem or blemished skin. Generally, however, the extract is obtained from linden blossoms and is credited with antiseptic, skin-clearing, soothing, sedative, circulation-stimulating, hydrating, and astringent properties. Linden extract may be used effectively in creams and emulsions for irritated skin, as well as in bath salts for the relaxation of muscle tension and cold.

linoleamide DEA—a highly effective thickener. It enhances product slip and feel and is also a conditioner, stabilizer, and viscosity builder. *See also* linoleic acid.

linoleamidopropyl PG-dimonium chloride phosphate—a vegetable-derived emulsifier. It leaves the skin with a smooth afterfeel. It is nonirritating.

linoleic acid (AKA vitamin F)—an emulsifier. Linoleic acid prevents dryness and roughness. A deficiency of linoleic acid in the skin is associated with symptoms similar to those characterizing eczema, psoriasis, and a generally poor skin condition. In numerous laboratory studies where a linoleic acid deficiency was induced, a topical application of linoleic acid in its free or esterified form quickly reversed this condition. In addition, linoleic acid is being found to inhibit melanin production in laboratory tests by decreasing tyrosinase activity and suppressing melanin polymer formation within melanosomes. Linoleic acid is an essential fatty acid found in a variety of plant oils, including soybean and sunflower.

linoleic acid ethylester—*see* ethyl linoleate.

linoleic acid triglyceride—an emollient. Not widely used because of its unsaturated nature that creates rancidity problems. It is a good penetrating agent.

linolenic acid—found in most drying oils. It is slightly irritating to the mucous membranes.

linolenic acid triglyceride—an emollient of limited use due to potential rancidity problems. It is a good penetrating agent.

linseed oil—botanical properties are listed as emollient, antiinflammatory, and healing. Derived from the flax plant seed, the oil is obtained by expression with little or no heat.

lipid concentrate—a vague description as it does not refer to the lipid's origin or source. Lipids, when added to the skin, are considered moisturizers. They renew the skin's barrier function and reduce moisture loss.

liposomes—double layer, hollow, spherical phospholipid membrane vesicles able to encapsulate water-soluble as well as oil-soluble substances (often proteins and peptides). Their structure and composition is similar to that of the skin. Their compatibility and affinity with cellular membranes allows them to be easily accepted and metabolized (as a lipid component) by the skin and provide the skin with "actives" that would not be so readily accepted otherwise. After much debate over their true efficacy and penetrating ability, it is now quite well established that the level of liposome effectiveness, measured in terms of their ability to deliver encapsulated "actives," is a function of the overall formulation technique and the liquid, gel, or cream in which the liposome is suspended. Empty or "unloaded" liposomes, as well as those loaded with emollients, can help reduce transepidermal water loss, thereby improving a dry skin condition and giving the skin smoothness. When containing linoleic acid, they can supply it to the sebaceous glands. It has been established that by remaining intact within the corneum layer, loaded liposomes may act as time releasers of valuable actives. When loaded with skin care agents, liposomes may assist in moisturizers by providing deeper levels of epidermal hydration. Filled with UV absorbers or antioxidants, such as superoxide dimutase (SOD) or the flavonoid type, liposomes are beneficial in sun protection formulations. In addition to their carrier abilities and penetration properties, liposomes leave the upper stratum corneum with a pleasant and smooth feeling. Liposomes are predominantly formed by phospholipids of natural, semisynthetic, and/or synthetic origin. Those of natural origin are obtained from yolk and soybean lecithin phospholipids. Liposomes are considered by some as revolutionary in the development of cosmetic concepts. They have brought to the cosmetic field widespread interest in the concepts of microencapsulation and targeted substance delivery.

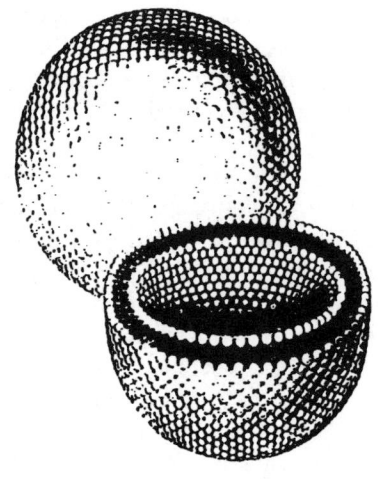

Liposomes

liquorice extract—*see* licorice extract.

liquorice root extract—*see* licorice extract.

live yeast cell derivative—*see* tissue respiratory factor.

lovage oil *(Levisticum officinale)*—ascribed botanical properties such as cleansing, depurative, and draining make lovage oil appropriate for use on oily skin. In addition, the roots and fruit have aromatic and stimulant activity. This oil is produced by distillation of the roots, though the leaves and seeds are also used for botanical purposes.

lysine—a skin-conditioning amino acid. *See also* amino acid.

lysine PCA—increases cellular oxygen intake and improves moisturization. Lysine PCA is also used as a neutralizing agent and pH buffer in skin care formulations.

lysine carboxymethyl cysteinate—a water-soluble amino acid complex with the ability to regulate oil secretion.

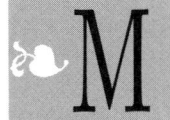

MI/MCI (AKA methylchloro isothiazolinone)—a preservative with high sensitizing potential in products intended to stay on the skin. Because of this its use is declining. Allergic reactions have been attributed to it, particularly in leave-on cosmetics such as night creams. Although the currently recommended concentration level ranges from 15 to 7.5 ppm (parts per million), MI/MCI in concentrations as low as 7 ppm may induce sensitization. It is generally advised that MI/MCI be used only in rinse-off products such as soaps and cleansers.

macadamia nut oil *(Macademia integrifolia)*—a carrier and an emollient with excellent spreadability and penetration properties. It leaves a good, smooth, nongreasy afterfeel and is very gentle to the skin. Its fatty acid composition is similar to the major fatty acid composition of skin sebum, including some of the acids that are crucial to the maintenance of the skin's water barrier functions. This oil is beneficial in products for mature and/or dry skins due to its palmitoleic oil content, which decreases in the skin over time. The oil is derived from the nuts of the macadamia tree, grown primarily in Australia and the Hawaiian Islands and closely related to the hazelnut. The nut's weight is 70 % oil, specifically a triglyceride oil with a large quantity of palmitoleic oil (22%). It is nonirritating to the eyes and has no known side effects.

Madonna lily—*see* white lily bulb extract.

magnesium—an important factor in various enzymatic processes. Magnesium plays a role in amino acid synthesis (the synthesis of proteins, including collagen) and in the metabolism of calcium, sodium, and phosphorus.

magnesium aluminum silicate—a thickener with texture-modification and emulsion-stabilizing abilities, as well as astringent properties. This is a refined and purified smectite clay. It is noncomedogenic and nontoxic.

magnesium laureth sulfate—a mild surfactant and cleansing agent.

magnesium sulfate—an inorganic salt used as a bulking agent in cosmetic preparations.

magnesium-1-ascorbyl-2-phosphate—a synthetic analogue to vitamin C. It is reported to be somewhat more stable and equally as effective as vitamin C in regulating collagen biosynthesis and as an antioxidant.

maize germ oil—*see* corn oil.

maize gluten amino acids—*see* corn amino acids.

maleated soya bean oil—*see* soybean oil.

mallow extract *(Malva sylvestris)*—anti-inflammatory, soothing, refreshing, and emollient properties are attributed to this ingredient. Mallow extract has a high mucilage content that, when in contact with water, swells and forms a soft, soothing, protective gel. It is beneficial in eye treatment preparations. In folkloric medicine, mallow extract was used for wound healing, and it was traditionally used in soothing treatments and dermatological disorders. The extract is often derived from the leaves and flowers of *Malva sylvestris*, generally known as blue, common, or high mallow, though it can be obtained from other types of mallow, such as marsh, musk, dwarf, and tree-sea.

malt extract—has rubefacient properties in cosmetics due to the presence of yeast. It is used in face masks and toning lotions as a nutrient and texturizer. Malt extract is a dark syrup obtained by evaporating an aqueous extract of partially germinated and dried barley seeds.

malva—a traditional emollient and moisturizer. Malva is part of the mallow family. *See also* mallow extract.

mammarian extract—a biological additive extracted from the bovine mammarian tissue. *See also* protein.

mandarine extract—has similar properties to those of orange extract. Obtained from mandarin orange peel. *See also* orange extract.

mandarin oil—its botanical properties are very close to those of orange, with mandarin's sedative and antispasmodic properties being more pronounced. Expressed from the peel of mandarin oranges.

manganese—a violet color. As an oligoelement, manganese plays a role in collagen synthesis and skin moisturizing. Patents have been assigned on the use of manganese, zinc, and copper in the treatment of acne and sunburns.

manganese aspartate—a chemical additive.

mannuronate methylsilanol—*see* methylsilanol mannuronate.

margosa oil—considered a healing oil for its antiseptic and sebum-regulating properties.

marigold extract *(Calendula officinalis)*—the general effects attributed to marigold extract include antiseptic, healing, and soothing. It is useful in eye treatment cosmetics. In addition, it may be beneficially used against sunburns and other superficial burns due to some emollient capabilities. Traditionally, marigold extract was used to heal skin rashes and cleanse little wounds after washing. Marigold extract's constituents include flavonoids, glycosides of oleanoic acid, carotenoids, and phenolic acid. The recommended usage level for this extract is 1–10%. The extract is obtained from the flowers.

marine plasma extract—may help in organizing the structure of connective tissue. It is considered healing due to its iodine content, which is present in a natural form complexed with algal peptides and polysaccharides. This makes it a more active and gentler product when applied to the skin. This extract contains plasma (the fluid part of the tissue from which suspend matter such as cells has been removed), vitamins, polysaccharides, essential sea minerals, and some cellular reagents. Trace minerals also include calcium, iron, magnesium, potassium, sodium, and silicon. Vitamin A, water-soluble vitamin B, vitamin C, pantothenic acid, and niacinamide are also present. Marine plasma extract is a trade name for a mixture comprised of a combination of brown algae and marine animals. It is obtained by extracting the liquid from the cellular mass of marine organisms. Not known to cause skin irritation.

marine seaweed extract—*see* algae extract; seaweed extract.

marine sediments—an all-encompassing name for a compound. *See also* algae extract; marine plasma extract; seaweed extract.

marjoram *(Origanum vulgare)*—described as tonic and antifungal. Although there are numerous species of marjoram, sweet marjoram and wild marjoram are the most popular for botanical applications. Similar properties are reported for both. *See also* marjoram oil.

marjoram oil—its ascribed botanical properties include antispasmodic, calming, and sedative indicating applications for sensitive or irritated skin. The oil is obtained through distillation. It may cause allergic reactions with symptoms being skin redness and itching.

marshmallow extract *(Althea officinalis)*—emollient and soothing. It can be pain relieving especially in the case of burns, sunburns, or scrapes. In traditional medicine, marshmallow extract was used as a local adjunct soothing and anti-itching agent for dermatological treatments. In folklore it has been used for rough skin, scruff, dry scabs, burns, scalds, and swelling. *See also* althea extract; mallow extract.

marshmallow root extract—*see* althea extract; marshmallow extract.

matricaria extract—an extract of the flowerheads of *Matricaria chamomilla*. *See also* chamomile extract.

meadowfoam oil *(Lamnanthes alba)*—a rich emollient. This mild, stable oil is resistant to oxidation. It is of much interest to cosmetic formulators because of its "dryness" and quick penetration into the skin. The oil is extracted from the meadowfoam seeds that contain 20–30% oil by weight.

meadowsweet extract *(Filipendula ulmaria* or *Spireae ulmaria)*—appears to have strong antifree radical properties, as well as analgesic and topical anti inflammatory activity. The anti-free radical activity is attributed to its flavonoid and tannin content, and the anti-inflammatory and analgesic properties are due to nonvolatile salicylate derivatives. Its analgesic, anti-inflammatory, and antifree radical activity make it particularly useful in suncare preparations. The word *aspirin* is derived from this plant's Latin name—a for acetyl and spirin from *Spireae*. Meadowsweet is a perennial plant that grows abundantly at the edges of rivers and ditches in meadows and damp woods.

medanione—used as a preservative in emollients. This is a synthetic ingredient with the properties of vitamin K. Used medically to prevent blood clotting.

melanin—a water-soluble form of melanin that can be formulated into a product as a free radical scavenger. Melanin can be naturally extracted from cuttle fish ink or synthetically produced. Research indicates that when employed as a sunscreen, melanin provides better UVA protection and requires lower usage concentrations than other available sunscreens. Its safety is supported through studies conducted with radioactive melanin, which showed no penetration through human skin.

melhydran—increases the skin's moisture-binding capacities. This is a honey derivative, specifically a concentrated and purified extract of Provence honey from thyme, lavender, and rosemary. It can also be produced synthetically.

melaleuca—*See* cajeput oil.

melilot *(Melilotus officinalis)* (AKA sweet clover; white clover)—credited with emollient, bactericidal, sedative, and virustatic properties. Traditionally, it was used on a couperose condition. Coumarin is melilot's only important constituent. Its related compounds are hydrocoumaric (melilotic) acid, orthocoumaric acid, and melilotic anhydride (lactone), which is a fragrant oil. There are several species of this perennial herb. The whole herb is used for botanical purposes.

melissa—*see* balm mint extract.

melissa oil—*see* balm mint oil.

menhaden oil—contains essential fatty acids vital to the metabolism of healthy skin. The oil is obtained from the small North Atlantic menhaden fish, which is a little larger than a herring.

menthol—a fragrance. It is also said to be antiseptic, cooling, refreshing, and a blood circulation stimulant. Menthol gives the skin a "cool" feeling after use. It constitutes almost 50% of peppermint oil but can also be made synthetically by hydrogenation of thymol. It is nontoxic in low doses, but in high concentrations it can be irritating to the skin and especially the mucous membranes. *See also* mint.

menthol extract—*see* menthol.

menthyl anthranilate—the only FDA-approved liquid sunscreen chemical with UVA absorption capabilities. It has an approved usage level of 3.5–5%. This is a stable ingredient and can be combined with other sunscreen chemicals to increase SPF while providing UVA protection.

menthyl lactate—a fragrance component. This is the ester of menthol and lactic acid.

mercaptopyridine—used in skin-lightening preparations due to its ability to retard melanin production and provide a skin-lightening effect.

mercurials—a preservative with a high sensitizing potential particularly in products intended to be left on the skin. Mercury is only used in minute amounts as a preservative in some eye makeup preparations to inhibit the growth of germs. Mercury is not for use in skin care formulations as it may cause a variety of symptoms ranging from chronic inflammation to fever and rash.

methicone—a type of silicone used primarily in the formulation of free-flowing cosmetic powders. Methicone can also be found in cosmetic preparations as a skin surface sealant to reduce transepidermal water loss.

methionin—*see* methionine.

methionine—slows down and normalizes oil gland sebum production. Methionine is also used as a texturizer in cosmetic creams. It is an essential amino acid found in a number of proteins and developed via fermentation.

methoxy PEG-22 dodecyl gylcol copolymer—an effective water-in-oil emulsifier with a high water-binding capability. This ingredient has good dermatological and toxicological properties and is very compatible with other skin care ingredients. This facilitates its incorporation into skin care preparations.

3,1-methoxypropane-1,2 diol—provides a cool sensation when used in facial masks.

methoxy propyl gluconamide—an alpha hydroxyacid derivative used as a moisturizer and an emollient. Its minimal acidity favors its use on dry and very dry, scaly skin surfaces where other alpha hydroxyacid compounds may not be well tolerated.

methyl gluceth-10—a skin humectant and a preservative. This is the polyethylene glcyol ether of methyl glucose.

methyl gluceth-20—a humectant skin-conditioning agent.

methyl glucose isostearate—an emulsifier with highly effective moisturizing properties.

methyl glucose sesquistearate—an emulsifier made from natural sources.

methyl hydroxy stearate—an emollient used in moisturizing formulations. This is the ester of methyl alcohol and hydroxystearic acid.

methyl paraben—one of the most frequently used preservatives because of its very low sensitizing potential. It is one of the oldest preservatives in use to combat bacteria and molds. Noncomedogenic.

methylchloroisothiazolinone—*see* MI/MCI.

methylisothiazolinone—a preservative. *See also* MI/MCI.

methylsilanol elastinate—a protein derivative used as a skin-conditioning agent.

methylsilanol hydroxyprolinate aspartate—classified as a skin-conditioning agent that can perform a number of different functions within a skin care formulation.

methylsilanol mannuronate—tests indicate that, as a result of its cutaneous hydration activity, it increases skin suppleness and moisturization and aids in the reduction of cellulite.

mica—used as a texturizer and coloring agent in cosmetics. Mica is the group name for a series of silicate minerals that are ground and have similar physical properties but vary their chemical composition. Micas vary in color from colorless to pale green, brown, or black.

microcrystalline cellulose—provides good slip and softness and acts as a binder. A cellulose fiber isolated from colloidal crystals. *See also* cellulose.

microcrystalline wax—an emulsifier. This is a beeswax substitute characterized by the fineness of its crystals (in comparison with the larger crystals of paraffin wax). It is derived from petroleum.

micronutrients—*see* trace elements.

milfoil extract *(Achillea millefolium)*—credited with antiseptic and antibiotic properties. *See also* yarrow extract.

milk protein—gives a smooth feel to the skin. Milk protein is primarily casein that is well absorbed by the skin and gives it gloss and fine touch by forming a soft film. It has a water-holding ability in the range of 13%. Milk protein is obtained from milk. If it is hydrolyzed, it is broken down into smaller pieces and is referred to either as hydrolyzed milk protein, milk amino acids, or casein amino acids.

milk thistle *(Carduus marianus)*—credited with wound healing. It is used in toners and aftershave preparations.

millerpertuis oil—used for sunburns, burns, and bruises.

mimosa bark extract—*see* mimosa tenuiflora.

mimosa essence—fragrance. Mimosa essence is credited with anti-inflammatory and astringent properties. It may produce allergic skin reactions. *See also* mimosa tenuiflora.

mimosa tenuiflora (AKA mimosa bark extract; *tepescohuite* [Mexican name])—used in cosmetics for its believed epidermic tissue regenerating, repairing, and protecting properties. It has also been described as a healing oil for its antiseptic properties. It can be used effectively in postsun preparations, baby skin care creams, and protective creams. Mimosa tenuiflora has a high bioflavonoid and tannin content that helps increase the skin's impermeability. This extract also contains zinc, necessary for DNA synthesis and cellular nutrition; iron, vital for oxygen transport and intracellular metabolism; magnesium, for its protective role; copper, for anti-inflammation; and manganese that is said to stimulate cellular metabolism. The mimosa tenuiflora tree, related to the acacia, is found only in Mexico's southeastern state of Chiapas. The bark is the part used. Mayan healers used bark powder on cutaneous lesions, and the Guatemalan inhabitants of the region still use it today. May produce allergic skin reactions.

mineral oil (AKA Russian white oil)—an emollient cleanser and demulsifier of dirt trapped in pores. Though widely used in European skin care products, its use is looked upon with distrust in the United States as many sources have classified it as comedogenic. Mineral oil is excellent for use in cleansers. In leave-on cosmetics its comedogenicity or lack thereof appears related to the level of raw material refinement; therefore some suppliers state that their product is noncomedogenic. When used in leave-on preparations, mineral oil's occlusive capability is considered to help improve the epidermal barrier function. This is a clear, odorless oil derived from petroleum and is not known to cause allergic reactions.

mineral pigments—provide UV protection. This refers to ingredients such as titanium dioxide or zinc oxide usually incorporated into sunscreens, makeup bases, and even daytime moisturizers to enhance the product's sunscreening ability or allow for truth behind a claim.

mineral wax—*see* ozokerite.

mink oil—a gentle and effective emollient with skin-softening abilities. Its occlusive properties give it skin-conditioning qualities as well. Obtained from the subdermal fatty tissues of the mink.

mint oil (*Mentha* sp.)—cooling, tonic, stimulating, antiseptic, and relaxing properties are attributed to mint. Mint was traditionally used as an adjunct soothing and anti-itching treatment in dermatological disorders. It has also been considered helpful for scratches and insect bites. In addition, this aromatic herb is widely used as a fragrance in beauty products. There are about 20 species in the *Mentha* genus growing around the world, including peppermint and spearmint—the two most widely used in skin care preparations. These serve as cleansers and decongestants indicated for acne and for dermatitis. Mint oil is produced by distillation of the plant.

mireth-3 myristate—an emollient employed as a skin-conditioning agent in cosmetic formulations.

mistletoe extract *(Phoradendron flavescens* and *Viscum album)*—antispasmodic, healing, and calming properties are attributed to this ingredient. Mistletoe is an evergreen, parasitic plant growing on tree branches where it forms pendent bushes 2 to 5 feet in diameter. The extract is obtained from the plant's berries.

monoammonium glycyrrhizinate—*see* glycyrrhizinate.

monomethylsilanetril lactate—an alpha hydroxyacid derivative with silicone.

monosodium n-cocoylglutamate—a surfactant.

montmorillonite—used as an abrasive in exfoliants and a bulking agent in masks. It is also used to increase a formula's viscosity and as an emulsion stabilizer and opacifying agent. Montmorillonite is a complex silicate. It is a clay mineral that forms the main ingredient of bentonite and Fuller's earth.

mucopolysaccharides—their strong moisture-binding capacity enhances a formulation's moisture-binding quality and reduces transepidermal water loss. Studies show that mucopolysaccharides will reduce the amount of moisture lost by the skin and will stimulate its moisture intake. This ingredient exhibits the desirable moisture-binding qualities of healthy skin giving the skin turgor, increased water content, and elasticity. Mucopolysaccharides are highly effective in skin treatment products. As a natural skin component, mucopolysaccharides fill the spaces between collagen and elastin protein fibers in the dermis, giving them support and providing lubrication and moisture.

mucoprotein (soluble)—*see* protein.

mucus of quince—*see* quince.

mud—a mixture of a powder and a liquid. Usually applied wet as a facial mask and allowed to dry. If the powder and/or liquid contain therapeutic ingredients, these will interact with the skin. Identifying this therapeutic action requires knowing the nature of the powder and liquid being used. In a mask, it also acts as an occlusive agent for the time the mask remains on the skin. This favors the interaction of ingredients in a cream or other product applied prior to the mud.

mulberry glycolic extract—astringent properties are attributed to this ingredient.

myristal myristate—an ester of myristyl alcohol and myristic acid. *See also* myristic acid; myristyl alcohol.

myristic acid—a surfactant and cleansing agent. When combined with potassium, myristic acid soap provides a very good, abundant lather. This is a solid organic acid naturally occurring in butter acids such as nutmeg, oil of lovage, coconut oil, mace oil, and most animal and vegetable fats. Although some sources site it as having no irritation potential, they do indicate a comedogenicity potential.

myristyl ether propionate—an emollient and skin-conditioning agent used in preshave lotions and moisturizing preparations.

myristyl alcohol—an emollient often used in hand creams, cold creams, and lotions to give them a smooth, velvety feel. Sources indicate it as being mildly comedogenic and with an irritancy potential.

myristyl lactate—a light emollient and moisturizer with good spreadability. It leaves a smooth, satiny afterfeel. Sources indicate it as being comedogenic and with a slight irritancy potential. *See also* lactic acid; myristyl alcohol.

myristyl myristate—an occlusive skin-conditioning agent useful in emulsions that have to "melt" once in contact with the skin. It gives good spreadability. This is an ester formed by the combination of the myristyl alcohol and myristic acid fractions of coconut oil. *See also* myristic acid; myristyl alcohol.

myristyl ocatanoate—a light emollient and moisturizer. It leaves the skin's surface with a smooth and supple finish.

myrrh extract *(Commiphora myrrah)*—said to have disinfectant, antiseptic, anti-inflammatory, anti-itching, cicatrizant, tonic, stimulant, sedative, and astringent properties. It is also a good fixative. Myrrh extract can be valuable in products designed for acne treatment. Myrrh is a traditional and ancient ingredient for perfumes and incense and was used by ancient Egyptian women in facial masks and other cosmetic preparations. Myrrh oil is produced by the distillation of the gum.

myrtle—astringent and antiseptic with botanical properties closely resembling those of eucalyptus. Indicated for acne and oily skin. Myrtle is obtained by distillation of the branches.

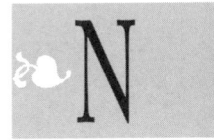

NaAl silicate—*see* sodium aluminum silicate.

nalidone—*see* pyrrolidonic carbon acid.

NaPCA—*see* sodium PCA.

narcissus flower extract—a fragrance. It has also been used as an antispasmodic. Recommended for use in very low concentrations as its oil has been shown to impair cellular functions when added to in vitro cell cultures. In addition, large amounts of the extract may produce headaches.

nasturtium extract *(Tropaeolum majus)*—considered to have disinfectant attributes, and be effective in acne treatment products. It is also said to have rubefactant properties. May produce allergic reactions.

natrium mud extract—*see* mud.

natural moisturizing factor (NMF)—refer to entry in chapter 4.

neem extract—may have insect-repellent properties.

neopentyl glycol dicaprate—an emollient also used to increase a formulation's viscosity. Primarily used in hand and body preparations.

neopentyl glycol dicaprylate/dicaprate—an emollient and formula viscosity-increasing agent used mostly in the manufacturing of lipsticks.

nerol—a primary alcohol used in perfumes, especially those with rose and orange blossom scents. Nerol is naturally occurring in oil of lavender, orange leaf, palmarosa oil, rose, neroli, and oil of petitgrain. It is colorless and has a roselike scent.

neroli—*see* neroli oil; orange flower oil.

neroli oil—a fragrance. It is used in skin care preparations to stimulate cell regeneration. Given its sedative and soothing properties, it is indicated for sensitive and delicate skin. However, neroli oil appears beneficial for all skin types. True neroli is extracted from bitter orange blossom. This is one of the most expensive oils and therefore is widely adulterated with the distillation of other citrus blossoms such as sweet orange, lemon, and mandarin. *See also* orange flower oil.

neroli water—*see* orange flower water.

nettle extract *(Urtica dioica)*—its botanical properties are listed as anti-inflammatory, astringent, bactericidal, healing, mildly deodorant, and stimulating. Some consider it effective for treating eczema and sunburn. According to some sources this is the botanical with the highest vitamin E content, and as such it would have good antioxidant properties. Nettle's important constituents include acetylcholine, amino acids, histamine, carotinoids, and chlorophyll. An analysis of fresh nettle also shows the presence of formic acid, mucilage, mineral salts, ammonia, carbonic acid, and water. The formic acid in nettle, along with the phosphates and a trace of iron, makes it a valuable botanical. There are more than 500 species of nettle growing mainly in tropical countries. The whole herb is employed for therapeutic purposes.

niacin—a skin-conditioning agent.

niacinamide (AKA vitamin B)—used as a skin stimulant. *See also* vitamin B.

niaouli oil—its therapeutic properties indicate possible improvement in circulation and antibody activity and healing in cases of infected wounds and burns. Some of its medicinal properties and indications are the same as those for eucalyptus. Niaouli oil is produced by distillation of the plant's leaves.

niosomes—nonionic surfactant vesicles similar to liposomes in structure. According to manufacturers, niosomes interact desirably with human skin when topically applied. They are prepared from suitable nonionic surfactants. *See also* liposomes.

nonfat dry milk—has soothing and moisturizing effects and is often used in facial masks. Nonfat dry milk consists mostly of protein and also contains lactic acid, lactose, vitamins, and minerals. *See also* milk protein.

nonoxynol—*see* polyoxyethylene nonylphenyl ether.

nonoxynol-14—a surfactant and emulsifying agent. It is used as a nonionic surface-active agent and as a dispersing agent in cosmetics.

norvaline—a protein amino acid used as a skin-conditioning agent. *See also* valeric acid.

nutmeg oil *(Myristica fragrans)*—credited with tonic and stimulating properties. Nutmeg oil is not commonly used in cosmetic formulations. The oil is produced by distillation of the nuts and can cause skin irritation.

nutrilan (AKA hydrolyzed animal protein)—creates a smooth, velvety feeling on the skin's surface. It contains amino acids present in the skin. Nutrilan is an example of how cosmetic companies can list their ingredients and create ambiguity with respect to identity or source. *See also* hydrolyzed animal protein.

nylon—a commonly known synthetic material used as a fiber in eyelash lengtheners and mascaras and as a molding compound to shape cosmetics. Nylon gives bulk to a compound and, when appropriate, provides opacifying properties. It can cause allergic reactions.

nylon 11—a bulking agent used primarily in makeup preparations and in some moisturizers.

nylon 12—a bulking and opacifying agent that provides good feel and good elasticity to moisturizers and makeup preparations, including foundations. A polyamide derivative of acid 12-aminododecanioic.

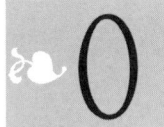

oak bark (*Quercus* sp.)—its botanical properties are described as slightly tonic, strongly astringent, and antiseptic. It also reduces inflammation and prevents infection. Its astringent effects were already well known centuries ago. Oak bark extract appears to have greater therapeutic effects than oak root.

oak bud extract—*see* aleppo gall.

oak root—exhibits soothing and anti-inflammatory properties. Oak root is recommended for sensitive skin, protecting it against unwanted reactions (e.g., swelling or redness). The extract is generally obtained from the younger part of the plant.

oakmoss empuree *(Evernia prunastri)*—a fragrance component derived from any one of several resin-yielding lichens that grow on oak trees.

oat *(Avena sativa)*—contains a colloid that has soothing properties on the skin. Generally speaking, all oat grades enhance emulsion stability, increase viscosity, leave a smooth afterfeel, and provide a source of whole natural vegetable protein. Oatmeal-based preparations are given by dermatologists for irritated skins resulting from sunburn, psoriasis, or allergic dermatitis. The oatmeal seems to both subdue the irritation and relieve redness and itching. It acts as a soap-free cleanser. Oats in the form of bran, flour, or meal provide a gentle base for face masks designed to work with delicate, sensitive skin. Oatmeal masks absorb oil from the skin's surface and reduce the redness of irritated, broken-out skin.

Oatmeal soaps are nonirritating and good for people with delicate, sensitive skin.

oat bran—*see* oat.

oat extract—an extract obtained from the seeds of oats. *See also* oat.

oat flour—an abrasive, absorbent, bulking, and viscosity-increasing substance obtained by the fine grinding of oat kernels. It is used in a variety of cosmetic preparations, including powders, masks, mudpacks, moisturizers, suntan gels, hand and body creams, and soaps. *See also* oat.

oat meal flour—used as an abrasive and bulking agent in paste masks and soaps. Obtained by grinding oats from which the husks have been removed. *See also* oat.

octadecanol—*see* stearic acid.

octadecene/maleic anhydride copolymer—an emulsion stabilizer, film former, and viscosity-increasing chemical used in cosmetic formulations.

octadodecyl stearyl stearate—an emollient.

octocrylene—a UVB sunscreen with strong water-resistant properties and a rather broad-band absorption range. This is an expensive ingredient that has a high minimum use percentage (7%). Although gaining some popularity among formulators, its expense and usage level limit acceptance and use.

octyl dimethyl PABA (AKA padimate-O; ρ-aminobenzoic acid)—an FDA-approved sunscreen chemical with an approved usage level of 1.4–8%. In the 1970s it was the most popular sunscreen chemical available, as it is one of the best UVB absorbers. Today it is being replaced by octyl-p-methoxycinnamate as a result of the PABA-free trend in sunscreen products. A PABA derivative, it can cause skin irritation. *See also* ρ-aminobenzoic acid.

octyldodecanol—formerly listed as octyl dodecanol. An emollient with good spreadability, this is a good vehicle for oil-soluble ingredients.

2-octyl-1-dodecanol—an emollient.

octyl methoxycinnamate (AKA ethylhexyl methoxycinnamate; ethylhexyl p-methoxycinnamate; 2-ethylhexyl p-methoxycinnamate)—an FDA-approved sunscreen chemical with an approved usage level of 2–7.5%. Currently this is the most popular sunscreen chemical incorporated worldwide into sun products. It has an excellent UV absorption capability, a good safety profile, broad solubility in oils, and insolubility in water. These attributes all add up to make it an almost perfect sunscreen chemical. Considered a noncomedogenic raw material, it is derived from balsam of Peru, cocoa leaves, cinnamon leaves, and storax. *See also* cinnamate.

octyl p-methoxycinnamate—*see* octyl methoxycinnamate.

octyl palmitate—a nongreasy, nonoily moisturizing ester with good spreadability and good solvency properties.

octyl pelargonate—a light emollient that does not leave a greasy feel on the skin.

octyl salicylate (AKA 2-ethylhexyl 2-hydroxybenzoate; 2-ethylhexyl salicylate)—an FDA-approved sunscreen chemical with an approved usage level of 3–5%. In suntan lotions it is also used as a preservative and antimicrobial. Its usage is gaining in popularity. Octyl salicylate is a salt of salicylic acid occurring in wintergreen leaves and other plants. Considered a noncomedogenic raw material. *See also* salicylic acid.

octyl stearate—an emollient with similar properties to those of octyl palmitate. *See also* stearic acid.

octyl triazone—an ultraviolet light absorber.

octylcrylene—*see* 2-ethylhexyl 2-cyano-3, 3-diphenylacrylate.

octyldodecanol—an emollient alcohol.

octyldodecyl benzoate—an emollient and a solvent with high spreadability. It leaves a pleasant feel on the skin.

octyldodecyl stearate—a noncomedogenic emollient.

octyldodecyl stearoyl stearate—a noncomedogenic skin-conditioning agent that provides occlusive properties. It is also used as a viscosity-increasing material in cosmetic formulations.

octyl hydroxystearate—an emollient used as a skin-conditioning agent.

old English walnut—*see* walnut.

oleamine—a chemical additive used in the formulation of cosmetics.

oleate sorbitan—*see* sorbitan oleate.

oleic acid—can improve the skin penetration abilities of a preparation's components. Obtained from various animal and vegetable fats and oils. Mildly irritating to the skin.

oleostearine—a mixture of the fatty acid triglycrides remaining after the physical separation of the low titre oils from beef tallow.

oleth 2—an emulsifier and solubilizer. This is a polyethylene glycol ether of oleyl alcohol. *See also* oleyl alcohol.

oleth 5—an emulsifier and solubilizer. It is also a spreading agent. *See also* oleyl alcohol.

oleth 10—a nonionic emulsifier and a solubilizer. *See also* oleyl alcohol.

oleth 20—a fragrance solubilizer especially useful in some clear gel systems. *See also* oleyl alcohol.

oleth 30—a surfactant used as a cleansing and solubilizing agent in cosmetic formulations. *See also* oleyl alcohol.

oleyl alcohol—an emollient, solvent, viscosity-increasing agent, and carrier employed in a wide variety of cosmetic formulations including makeup, skin care, and hand and body preparations. Oleyl alcohol is an unsaturated fatty alcohol found in fish oils and can also be produced synthetically. According to some sources it is comedogenic and has a mild irritancy potential.

oleyl betaine—a mild emollient, conditioning surfactant, and formulation thickener. *See also* betain; oleamine.

oleyl erucate—an all-purpose emollient sometimes used as a jojoba oil substitute.

olibanum—*see* frankincense.

olibanum oil—a fragrance component. It is astringent with slight anti-inflammatory properties. *See also* frankincense.

oligo active liposomes—liposomes encapsulated with oligo-elements.

oligoelements—refer to entry in chapter 4. *See also* trace elements.

olive oil *(Olea europaea)*—a carrier oil with excellent lubricity, pale color, and low odor. Olive oil is considered an especially good carrier for essential oils. Its unsaponifiable fraction is described also as a type of precursor, though not a biological one, with some claims of its targeting epidermal keratinocytes and stimulating the synthesis of such substances as collagen, elastin, proteoglycans, and glycoproteins.

orange essence—used for fragrance.

orange oil (*Citrus aurantium* [bitter orange] and *Citrus sinensis* [sweet orange])—primarily used in perfumery. Its botanical properties in skin care are considered antispasmodic and sedative, making it suitable for sensitive, delicate skin.

orange flower extract—used in folk medicine as a mild sedative. It is considered effective for dry skin. *See also* orange flower oil.

orange flower oil—a fragrance. Credited with soothing and calming properties when used in skin care preparations. Orange flower oil should not to be confused with orange flower extract. The flowers from the bitter orange tree yield, by distillation, an essential oil known as neroli, which forms one of the principal elements of eau de cologne. A pomade and an oil are also obtained from orange flowers via maceration. The oil from sweet orange blossoms is far less fragrant than that from bitter orange. The flowers are distilled immediately after being gathered. The essential oil, which rises to the surface of the distillate, is drawn off, while the aqueous portion is sold as orange flower water. One hundred kilograms of flowers will yield 600 grams of oil by volatile solvents, 400 grams by the maceration method, and only 100 grams by enfleurage. Obtained by extraction or pressing of orange skin.

orange flower water—has similar properties to orange oil, but its soothing properties appear to be more pronounced. *See also* orange flower oil.

orange roughy oil—in skin care preparations it demonstrates superior spreading and skin-softening properties. A fish oil.

orchid extract (*Orchis* sp.)—enjoys a widespread reputation as a restorative and rejuvenator, apparently due more to the beauty of the flower than to any specific stimulant properties. Some sources credit it as good for dry skin but fail to cite why. The extract is obtained from the tubers of various orchid species.

orizanol (AKA orysanol)—a protector from UV radiation with an antioxidizing effect on fats and oils. Orizanol is a powder obtained from rice germ oil.

orysanol—*see* orizanol.

ovarian extract—a biological additive derived from bovine ovaries.

oxybenzone (AKA benzophenone-3)—an FDA-approved sunscreen chemical with an approved usage level of 2–6% and classified as a UVA absorber. Oxybenzone enhances SPF and is popular among sunscreen formulators. Considered a noncomedogenic raw material.

oxyquinoline sulfate—a disinfectant and a preservative against fungus growth. Made from phenols.

ozokerite (AKA cresin)—a microcrystalline wax found in the earth. It regulates formulation viscosity, has suspension properties, and gives products stability. Ozokerite is a hydrocarbon wax derived from mineral or petroleum sources that, upon refining, yields a hard white microcrystalline wax known as cresin.

P

PABA—*see* ρ-aminobenzoic acid.

padimate A—*see* amyldimethyl PABA.

padimate O—*see* octyl dimethyl PABA.

palm oil (hydrogenated)—used as a consistency regulator and a formula stabilizer in the manufacture of creams, lotions, makeup, and decorative cosmetics.

palm oil glycerides (hydrogenated)—used as a co-emulsifier, dispersing agent, and consistency regulator in the manufacture of cosmetics. It imparts a pleasant skin feel.

palm kernel glycerides (hydrogenated)—an emulsifier and consistency regulator. It is a mixture of mono-, di-, and triglycerides derived from palm kernel oil.

palm kernel oil—used primarily for making soaps and ointments. It is a natural oil obtained from the kernel of *Elaeis guineensis*.

palmkernelamide DEA—used as a nonionic surfactant, thickener, foam booster, and formula stabilizer in cosmetic preparations.

palmarosa oil *(Cymbopogon martini)*—properties attributed to this oil are soothing, moisturizing, antiseptic, and cell regeneration. Its use is indicated for acne skin and dermatitis condition as well as for dry skin. Palmarosa oil is said to have immediate calming and refreshing action on the skin. Widely used in perfumery and cosmetology,

231

palmarosa oil's fresh, roselike scent makes it useful for the adulteration of rose oil, one of the most expensive essential oils. The oil is obtained by distillation of the herb.

palmitic acid—employed as a formula texturizer. This acid is naturally occurring in allspice, anise, calamus oil, cascarilla bark, celery seed, butter acids, coffee, tea, and many animal fats and plant oils. It is obtained from palm oil, Japan wax, or Chinese vegetable tallow.

pancreatic enzymes—certain pancreatic enzymes (e.g., kallikrein), generally extracted from swine and/or bovine pancreas glands, can act as vasodilators when used in topically applied cosmetics. They are reported to improve cell mitosis, wound healing, and oxygen uptake and protect from UV radiation. Pancreatic enzymes are said to increase cell permeability thereby enhancing cellular absorption of nutrients. Another pancreatic enzyme, pancreatin, contains several enzymes that give it proteolytic, amylolytic, and lipolytic activity. It is used as a raw material in biological exfoliants to help remove cells from the corneum layer.

pansy extract *(Viola tricolor)*—its botanical properties include soothing, healing, and cleansing. Pansy extract is recommended for use in dry skin preparations and for skin problems of various types. This extract contains salicylic acid.

panthenol (AKA vitamin B$_5$)—acts as a penetrating moisturizer. Although the exact mechanism is unknown, panthenol appears to stimulate cellular proliferation and aid in tissue repair. Studies indicate that, when topically applied, panthenol penetrates the skin and is converted into pantothenic acid, a B complex vitamin. Such action could possibly influence the skin's natural resources of pantothenic acid. It imparts a nonirritant, nonsensitizing, moisturizing, and conditioning feel and promotes normal keratinization and wound healing. Panthenol protects the skin against sunburn, provides relief for existing sunburn, and enhances the natural tanning process. Its humectant character enables panthenol to hold water in the product or attract water from the environment, resulting in a moisturizing effect. As a skin softener it provides suppleness, and claims are that it also acts as an anti-inflammatory agent. Considered a noncomedogenic raw material.

panthenyl triacetate—a panthotenic acid derivative with vitamin B activity. *See also* pantothenic acid.

pantothenic acid—part of the vitamin B complex. It is considered a biological precursor capable of acting as a bioactivator. Pantothenic acid's relatively small molecule facilitates permeation of the epidermis, allowing it to participate in the metabolic process of the dermis. It is found in liver, eggs, dried brewer's yeast, and royal jelly.

papain—a papaya enzyme with the ability to dissolve keratin. Papain is used in face masks and peeling lotions as a very gentle exfoliant. Papain can be irritating to the skin but is less so than bromelin, a similar enzyme found in pineapples and also used in cosmetics. Considered a noncomedogenic raw material.

papaya *(Carica papaya)*—considered a cleanser for skin with acne condition. Its value resides in its papain enzyme content. *See also* papain.

papaya enzyme—*see* papain.

parabens—one of the most commonly used group of preservatives in the cosmetic, pharmaceutical, and food industries. Parabens provide bacteriostatic and fungistatic activity against a diverse number of organisms and are considered safe for use in cosmetics, particularly in light of their low sensitizing potential. An evaluation of preservatives for use in leave-on cosmetic preparations lists parabens among the least sensitizing. The range of concentrations used in cosmetics varies between 0.03–0.30% depending on the conditions for use and the product to which the paraben is added.

paraffin—used in cosmetics as a beeswax substitute. Paraffin is a solid mixture of hydrocarbons obtained from petroleum, though it can also be obtained from wood or coal. Pure paraffin is harmless to the skin, but the presence of impurities may result in irritation, eczemas, and other skin problems.

parsley extract *(Petroselinum sativum)*—serves as a deodorant. It is said to have disinfectant and anti-inflammatory properties.

parsley oil—traditionally used for soothing and anti-itching treatment in dermatological disorders. It may also be used as a preservative. Parsley oil is extracted from the seeds that contain an oil called apiol. It may cause allergic reactions in sensitive skin.

parsley seed—*see* parsley oil.

partially hydrolyzed protein—*see* protein.

passion flower extract *(Passiflora incarnata)*—botanical properties are described as antispasmodic and calming. Its active principle, passiflorine, appears to be somewhat similar to morphine.

passion fruit extract—an emollient with moisturizing and refreshing properties. Some of its most important constituents include vitamins, polysaccharides, minerals, and amino acids. This extract has an aromatic, fruity, tropical scent.

passion fruit oil—seen most often on sun care product labels, probably for a marketing effect due to the tropical connotation of passion fruit.

patchouli lite oil—*see* patchouli oil.

patchouli oil *(Pogostemon patchouli)* (AKA patchouly)— botanical properties are described as astringent, anti-inflammatory, and decongestive. Other properties are listed as tonic, stimulant in low doses, and sedative at high doses. Its botanical attributes make it useful also for acne, aged and chapped skin, and skin redness. In the Orient it was a renowned antidote against insect and snake bites. Also used as a perfume in soaps and cosmetics to impart a long-lasting oriental aroma. This oil has a strong, sweet, musty, and very persistent fragrance. The patchouli leaves are dried and fermented prior to distillation. May produce an allergic reaction in sensitive individuals.

patchouly—*see* patchouli oil.

PCA (AKA Ajidew; Ajidew A-100; 2-pyrrolidone-5-carboxylic acid)—PCA is quite hygroscopic and serves as a fine humectant. It is frequently used as a moisturizer.

peach extract *(Prunus persica)*—the bark and leaves are credited with curative powers. Herbalists have credited extracts made of peach leaves with the ability to help stop bleeding and heal wounds. Peach extract is recommended for use in products for dry skin.

peach oil—a carrier oil. *See also* peach extract; peach kernel oil.

peach kernel oil—a carrier credited with calming and soothing properties. This oil is expressed from the peach kernels.

peach stones (ground)—used in scrubs as exfoliants.

peanut fat—used to add consistency to cosmetic products. Peanut fat is hydrogenated peanut oil. *See also* peanut oil.

peanut oil—utilized as a skin softener, emulsifier, and emollient. It can also be used as a substitute for more expensive oils such as almond and olive in cosmetic creams. Peanut oil has a higher vitamin A, vitamin E, and nicotinic acid content than other nut oils. Peanut oil is obtained by pressing of the seed kernels and is harmless to the skin.

pectin—used as a thickening agent in cosmetic preparations due to its gelling properties. It is soothing and mildly acidic. Extracted from apples or the inner portion of citrus fruit rind.

PEG—the acronym for polyethylene glycol. Refer to PEG entry in chapter 4.

PEG 4—a binder, plasticizing agent, solvent, and softener. It improves resistance to moisture and oxidation. This ethylene oxide polymer is used primarily in hair products.

PEG 8—a humectant, binder, solvent, and viscosity modifier. Depending on source and molecular weight, it can be effectively used as a moisture and consistency regulator in creams, lotions, shaving preparations, and leave-on hair care products.

PEG 14—a humectant and solvent.

PEG 20—a humectancy and solvency agent used in suntan preparations, moisturizers, and cleansing products.

PEG 75—a binder, humectant, and solvent used in hair and skin care formulations.

PEG 100—a binder, humectant, and solvent.

PEG 200—a binder, humectant, and solvent.

PEG 7M—a binder, emulsion stabilizer, and viscosity-increasing agent used primarily in soaps and cleansing products.

PEG 6 beeswax—a surfactant-emulsifying agent that can gelate lipids.

PEG 8 beeswax—*see* PEG 6 beeswax.

PEG 12 beeswax—*see* PEG 6 beeswax.

PEG 20 beeswax—*see* PEG 6 beeswax.

PEG-6 caprylic/capric glycerides—an emollient and emulsifying agent that helps preserve the skin's lipid content and keep the skin soft. Studies indicate good effectiveness in psoriasis treatment due to its ability to soften the scaling skin and improve the action of the active ingredient being applied. Manufacturer test results indicate no primary toxic or allergic reactions and good skin tolerance.

PEG 30 castor oil—an emollient, detergent, emulsifier, and oil-in-water solubilizer recommended for fragrance oils and other oils that may be difficult to solubilize.

PEG 30 castor oil (hydrogenated)—*see* PEG 30 castor oil.

PEG 40 castor oil—a surfactant and powerful solubilizer used for solubilizing essential oils and perfumes in oil-in-water creams and lotions. It is similar to PEG 30 castor oil but more dense—a soft paste rather than a liquid.

PEG 40 castor oil (hydrogenated)—a nonionic emulsifier and solubilizer for essential oils and perfumes.

PEG 18 castor oil dioleate—an emulsifier for creams and lotions and a viscosity-increasing agent. It is particularly suitable when animal and vegetable oils are used.

PEG 2 ceteareth—an emulsifier.

PEG 6 dioleate—a surfactant-emulsifying agent derived from oleic acid. Used as a carrier or base in lotions and other cosmetic preparations.

PEG 150 distearate—a surfactant used as a cleansing and solubilizing agent.

PEG 7 glyceryl cocoate—a self-emulsifying emollient especially suitable for aqueous formulations.

PEG 60 glycerylisostearate—a surfactant-emulsifying agent.

PEG 5 glyceryl stearate—a surfactant-emulsifying agent used in moisturizing and cleansing products.

PEG 50 lanolin—a surfactant used as a cleansing and solubilizing agent primarily in hair straighteners. A lanolin derivative.

PEG 75 lanolin—an emollient, emulsifier, dispersant, plasticizer, and foam stabilizer. A polyethylene glycol derivative of lanolin.

PEG 75 lanolin oil—a surfactant used as a cleansing and solubilizing agent primarily in hair care products. Some use it in soap and cleanser formulations. A derivative of lanolin oil.

PEG 85 lanolin—a surfactant.

PEG 2 methyl ether—*see* dipropylene glycol monomethyl ether.

PEG 120 methyl glucose dioleate—a cleansing agent used in soaps, cleansers, and shampoos.

PEG octanoate—all PEG octanoates are listed as emulsifying agents regardless of the number of PEGs in the formulation.

PEG 20 oleate—an emulsifier derived from oleic acid.

PEG 25 PABA—an ultraviolet light absorber derived from PABA.

PEG 45 palm kernel glycerides—an emollient and emulsifying agent derived from palm kernel glycerides.

PEG 40 ricinoleyl ether—*see* ricinoleth 40.

PEG 10 sorbitan laurate—a cleansing and solubilizing agent. This is one of the most popularly used PEGs. PEG sorbitan laurates are very popular because of their mildness and therefore are used in a variety of preparations, including cosmetics, suntan products, toiletries, and fragrances. As a group they are considered noncomedogenic raw materials.

PEG 40 sorbitan laurate—a cleansing and solubilizing agent. *See also* PEG 10 sorbitan laurate.

PEG 44 sorbitan laurate—a cleansing and solubilizing agent. *See also* PEG 10 sorbitan laurate.

PEG 75 sorbitan laurate—a cleansing and solubilizing agent. *See also* PEG 10 sorbitan laurate.

PEG 80 sorbitan laurate—a cleanser and solubilizing agent considered a good anti-irritant. *See also* PEG 10 sorbitan laurate.

PEG 3 sorbitan oleate—an emulsifying agent. Commonly used in cosmetic, toiletry, and fragrance preparations and suntan gels.

PEG 6 sorbitan oleate—an emulsifying agent. *See also* PEG 3 sorbitan oleate.

PEG 3 sorbitan stearate—an emulsifying agent and a popular PEG among cosmetic formulators for use in all cosmetic, toiletry, and fragrance preparations, including suntan gels.

PEG 6 sorbitan stearate—an emulsifying agent. *See also* PEG 3 sorbitan stearate.

PEG 60 sorbitan stearate—an emulsifying agent. *See also* PEG 3 sorbitan stearate.

PEG 5 soya sterol—an emollient, emulsifier, and emulsion stabilizer. It is a derivative of sterols found in soybean oil and is considered a noncomedogenic raw material.

PEG 10 soya sterol—an emollient, viscosity modifier, and emulsifier used in a wide variety of skin and hair care products. It is derived from soybean oil.

PEG stearate—all PEG stearates are emulsifying agents. Some are more frequently used or are more suitable for use in particular types of preparations, such as body creams and lotions versus cleansers.

PEG 2 stearate—an emulsifier for creams and lotions. This tan-colored wax is derived from stearic acid. *See also* PEG stearate.

PEG 5 stearate—listed as particularly applicable for hand and body lotions and creams. *See also* PEG stearate.

PEG 6 stearate—used primarily as an emulsifier in the formulation of cleansing products. *See also* PEG stearate.

PEG 32 stearate—a cleansing and solubilizing agent often used in face and neck preparations as well as moisturizers. *See also* PEG stearate.

PEG 8 stearate—an emulsifier and thickening agent generally incorporated into hair care products, hand and body creams, and moisturizing preparations. Also a superfattening agent for shaving preparations and foam baths. *See also* PEG stearate.

PEG 30 stearate—a cleansing and solubilizing agent often suitable for moisturizing preparations. *See also* PEG stearate.

PEG 40 stearate—a hydrophilic emulsifier, stabilizer, antigellant, and lubricant for skin care formulations. Tends to be incorporated into a variety of skin care products and some hair care preparations, toiletries, and perfumes. *See also* PEG stearate.

PEG 100 stearate—a stabilizer and emulsifier for creams and lotions. Technically it is the polyethylene glycol ester of stearic acid containing 100 moles of PEG. It is also a cleansing agent and surfactant utilized in skin care products, some hair care preparations, toiletries, and some perfumes. *See also* PEG stearate.

pentaerythrityl stearate/caprate/caprylic adipate— an extremely emollient compound with moisturizing and protective properties. It is also a viscosity-building agent.

pentasodium pentate—an inorganic salt used as a water softener, emulsifier, and sequestering and dispersing agent in cleansing creams and lotions. Prepared from the dehydration of mono- and disodium phosphates. It is moderately irritating to the skin and mucous membranes.

peony extract *(Paeonia officinalis)*—clinical studies show peony extract to help improve acne condition and some skin diseases.

peppermint *(Mentha piperita)*—in extract form it helps relieve skin irritation and itching. It reduces skin redness due to inflammation or acne, cools by constricting capillaries, and has refreshing and tonic properties.

peppermint oil—credited with refreshing, cooling, bactericidal, and anti-irritant properties. It is also used as a fragrance. Peppermint oil can produce allergic reactions such as hay fever, skin rashes, and irritation, especially if a dressing is applied over the oil. Extracted from the leaves of the peppermint plant, menthol accounts for more than 50% of its content. *See also* mint oil.

peptide—*see* protein.

peptone—*see* protein.

perfluoropolyether—a liquid polymer able to form a protective and lubricating film on the skin. Recommended as a skin protectant against aggressive chemicals such as surfactants, alkalis, and organic solvents. It is suitable for dry and oily skins due to its lipo and hydrophobic properties. This ingredient also enhances product stability and improves product feel on the skin.

perfluoropolymethylisopropylether—used in formulations to stabilize emulsions, reduce skin moisture loss, and provide a product with a silky feel.

perhydroxysqualene (AKA squalane)—an emollient that can be obtained from a variety of sources, including wheat germ, olive and bran oils, and shark liver oil. When obtained from shark liver oil it must be converted from squalene through a process of hydrogenization.

petit grain biguarade—*see* petit grain oil.

petit grain extract—credited with tonic and antiseptic properties. *See also* petit grain oil.

petit grain oil (AKA petitgrain)—widely used in pharmacy and perfumery for its therapeutic and tonic effect. Its fragrance is fresh, invigorating, and slightly floral with a bitter note. Like neroli, real petitgrain (or petitgrain biguarade) is obtained by distilling the leaves of the bitter orange tree. Petitgrain bergamot, petitgrain lemon, and petitgrain mandarin are also produced. May be irritating to the skin.

petitgrain—*see* petit grain oil.

petrolatum (AKA petroleum jelly; Vaseline)—softens and smooths the skin. It forms a film on the skin's surface, preventing moisture loss due to evaporation and protecting against irritation. Its disadvantage lies in the difficulty of effectively and properly removing it from the skin. Studies conducted in 1992 indicate that petrolatum accelerates the recovery of skin surface lipids. It was also indicated that petrolatum neither forms nor acts as an impermeable membrane. Rather, it permeates throughout the corneum layer, allowing normal barrier recovery despite its occlusive properties. Petrolatum imparts a more greasy feeling than other emollients and also has the potential for clogging pores and causing comedogenicity. It is a purified mixture of semisolid hydrocarbons from petroleum. Although it can cause allergic skin rashes, petrolatum is nontoxic to the skin when properly purified and of high grade.

petroleum jelly—*see* petrolatum.

phenethyl alcohol—*see* phenylethyl alcohol.

phenol—frequently used for chemical face peels. It may trap free radicals and can act as a preservative. Phenol, however, is an extremely caustic chemical with a toxicity potential. It is considered undesirable for use in cosmetics. Even at low concentrations it frequently causes skin irritation, swelling, and rashes.

L-phenylalanine—an amino acid used as a skin-conditioning agent. It has greater use in hair care than in skin care products.

phenoxyethanol—a broad-range preservative with fungicidal, bactericidal, insecticidal and germacidal properties. It has a relatively low sensitizing factor in leave-on cosmetics. Phenoxyethanol can be used in concentrations of 0.5–2.0% and in combination with other preservatives such as sorbic acid or the parabens. It can also be used as a solvent for aftershaves, face and hair lotions, shampoos, and skin creams of all types. It can be obtained from phenol.

phenoxyethylparaben—a preservative considered a non-comedogenic raw material.

2-phenyl-5-benzimidazolesulfonic acid—*see* phenylbenzimidazole sulfonic acid.

phenyl dimethicone—an antifoaming agent and an occlusive skin-conditioning agent. This mixture of linear siloxane polymers is a silicone-derived material. *See also* dimethicone.

phenyl trimethicone—serves as a barrier protecting the skin from excessive water loss. It leaves the skin feeling soft and smooth, adds emolliency to the formulation, and reduces its feeling of tackiness. It is a form of silicone, similar to dimethicone but with a broader range of compatibility with organic oils and waxes.

phenylalanine—a conditioning agent with greater application in hair care than in skin care preparations. It is also used in suntan products.

phenylbenzimidazole sulfonic acid (AKA 2-phenyl-5-benzimidazolesulfonic acid; 2-phenylbenzimidazole-5-sulfonic acid)—one of 21 FDA-approved sunscreen chemicals for UVB absorption. It has an approved usage level of 1–4%. When combined with a proper base it becomes a water-soluble sunscreen. It exhibits a very effective use level versus SPF relationship when compared to other sunscreen chemicals. In addition, when combined with other UVB absorbers it seems to significantly boost SPF. Also excellent for use in clear sunscreen gels. Its performance is not completely understood.

2-phenylbenzimidazole-5-sulfonic acid (AKA 2-phenyl-5-benzimidazolesulfonic acid)—*see* phenylbenzimidazole sulfonic acid.

phenylethyl alcohol (AKA phenethyl alcohol)—has disinfectant and preservative properties and is also employed as a fragrance. It is a primary component of rose oil and is also found in oranges, raspberries, and tea.

phosphatides—*see* phospholipids.

phospholipids (AKA phosphatides)—used topically as a moisture/emollient because of their inherent compatibility with skin lipids. In general, natural phospholipids have a short-lived effect when topically applied and are a primary material in the manufacture of liposomes. Phospholipids are complex fat substances that, together with protein, form the membrane of all living cells. *See also* liposomes.

phosphatidic acid—one of several minor components of cosmetic and pharmaceutical liposomal membranes.

phosphatidylcholine—a major component of most cosmetic and pharmaceutical liposome structures, derived from commercially available egg yolk or soybean lecithin.

phosphatidyl ethanolamine—a minor component of cosmetic and pharmaceutical liposomal membranes.

phosphatidylinositol—a minor component of cosmetic and pharmaceutical liposomal membranes.

phosphatidylserine—used as an amphiphilic component in the manufacturing of large quantities of liposomes.

phosphoenolpyruvic acid—skin care preparations containing this ingredient are said to improve dry skin due to its moisturizing properties and its ability to accelerate cell turnover.

phosphoric acid—a preservative and an antioxidant. It is irritating to the skin in concentrated solutions.

phytosterol oleate—the prefix phyto- means plant. *See also* sterols.

pigskin extract—the extract of the skin of young pigs. *See also* protein.

pine extract (*Pinus* sp.)—the different varieties of pine yield resin in greater or smaller quantities, of which a very small amount is employed for therapeutic purposes, primarily as ointments. Pine's therapeutic properties are described as bactericidal and stimulating to blood circulation. Manufacturers usually specify if the extract is from the pine's bark, cone, or needle. Can be irritating to the skin and cause red splotches.

pine bark extract—used as a solvent. It is also an antiseptic and stimulant. Pine bark extract can cause skin irritation.

pine cone extract—said to be a skin stimulant. This extract is obtained from pine cones. *See also* pine extract.

pine needle extract—recommended for use as a skin stimulant. It is the extract of the needles of various pine species.

pine oil—originally used as a solvent and a disinfectant. Studies are now showing that pine oil may stimulate the growth of fibroblasts, which would mean an increase in the turnover of epidermal cells. Pine oil is produced by distillation of small pine branches. It may be irritating to the skin and mucous membranes.

pineapple enzyme—used in folkloric medicine as an anti-inflammatory. It is currently used in face masks and peeling lotions to remove the top layers of cells. Pineapple's activity is based on bromelin, an enzyme that dissolves keratin. Its important constituents include mucins, amino acids, polysaccharides, minerals, flavonoids, and enzymes. It can be irritating to the skin.

piscine oil/C30–C46—a fish oil used as an emollient.

placenta extract—claimed to increase skin's oxygen absorption, stimulate cell metabolism, and accelerate cellular reproductive activity when incorporated into a skin care preparation. Placenta extracts contain many vitamins and female hormones that, under certain circumstances, have been shown to help the appearance of aging skin. There is a question, however, as to how much vitamin or specific hormone is present in a given placenta-containing cream. The FDA requires that the concentration of vitamins and hormones in any such product be listed, but cosmetics containing placenta do not tend to list these. Scientists maintain that no evidence has been presented to substantiate the skin benefit claims made with respect to this ingredient. The placenta extract used in the United States is derived from bovine placenta.

placenta oil extract—*see* placenta extract.

placenta protein (bovine)—the protein derived from bovine placenta. *See also* placenta extract.

plant extracts—an all-encompassing and vague term usually used for marketing effect. Its lack of specificity does not allow for the identification of potential benefits, botanical properties, or irritating effects.

plantain extract (*Plantago* sp.)—credited with cooling, soothing, antiseptic, astringent, and bacteriostatic botanical properties. It is a bananalike fruit.

plantain fruit—*see* banana oil.

pollen extract—an extract of flower pollen.

poloxamer 188—a liquid surfactant polymer.

poloxamer 788—a surfactant polymer. A change in number (e.g., poloxamer 188 versus poloxamer 788) indicates the consistency of the ingredient, generally from liquid to paste to solid. The higher the number, the more solid the consistency.

polyacrylamide—a binder, film former, and fixative with greater use in hair and nail than in skin care preparations. It is used in some hand and body lotions and cleansing creams. It is prepared from acylonitirile and is toxic and irritating to the skin.

polyacrylic acid salt—a binder, emulsion stabilizer, film former, and viscosity-increasing agent primarily used in shampoos.

polyalkoxy ester—a thickener, auxiliary emulsifier, and body agent in cosmetic formulations.

polybutene—a binder and viscosity-increasing agent used more in makeup than skin care preparations. Polybutene is a polymer of one or more butylenes obtained from petroleum oils.

polybutylene terephthalate—a film former and viscosity-increasing agent.

polyethylene—used to regulate viscosity, suspension properties, and general stability in cosmetic formulations. It is derived from petroleum gas or dehydration of alcohol.

polyethylene beads—used in scrubs as replacement for almond particles. Some companies prefer it as they consider it less abrasive for delicate skins.

polyethylene glycol (AKA PEG)—a binder, solvent, plasticizing agent, and softener widely used for cosmetic cream bases and pharmaceutical ointments. PEGs are quite humectant up to a molecular weight of 500. Beyond this weight their water uptake diminishes.

polyethylene particles—*see* polyethylene beads.

polyethylene terephthalate—a film former and viscosity-increasing agent. This is a synthetic polymer.

polyglucadyne —*see* polyglucan.

polyglucan (AKA beta-glucan; polyglucadyne)—a new ingredient reported to enhance the skin's natural defense mechanism, which becomes less effective with age and exposure to UV light. It is also credited with wound-healing properties and it promotes cellular activity; serves as a topical moisturizer with long-lasting moisturizing effects; reduces wrinkles; helps protect the skin from infection; and protects the skin from invasion by toxic agents caused by pollution and injuries due to abrasions, exposure to UV light, extremes in climatic conditions, etc. In addition to this impressive list, polyglucans are also credited with immunostimulatory properties. A polyglucan is a hydrophilic ingredient, able to absorb more than 10 times its weight in water. It can be absorbed into the outer layers of the epidermis due to its extremely small size, thereby facilitating penetration into the pores and follicular openings of the skin. Once applied on the skin it forms a protective, hydrated film with excellent adhesive properties that do not appear to interfere with normal skin respiration. These film-forming and protective properties are particularly valuable for aging skin suffering from diminished collagen and elastin as well as impaired hydration and elasticity. Derived from yeast cell walls, polyglucans are compatible for formulation with all normally used skin care and other cosmetic ingredients. *See also* glucans.

polyglyceryl-3-dioleate—an emulsifier for water-in-oil emulsions. Listed as being very suitable for use in baby care products, water-resistant sun-protection products, skin creams, and dry skin treatment products. It is an ester of oleic acid with polyglycerol.

polyglyceryl-10 dipalmitate —*see* decaglyceryl dipalmitate.

polyglycerylmethacrylate—a film former used in moisturizers, skin care products, and fragrance preparations. It is a synthetic polymer.

polyglyceryl-4-oleate—used as an emulsifier in cosmetic formulations. It may also be used as a lubricant, plasticizer, gelling agent, and dispersant. It is prepared by adding alcohol to coconut oil or other triglycerides.

polymethylacrylate—serves as a film former. It is a synthetic polymer used in suntan gels, creams, and liquids as well as a variety of makeup preparations such as blushes, foundations, and powders.

polymethoxy bicyclic oxazolidine—a preservative active against yeast, bacteria, and mold. It can be used alone or with parabens, in which case it contributes to the preservative activity. This ingredient can be used in rinse-off and leave-on cosmetics with manufacturers reporting a good toxicological profile at recommended use levels.

polyols stearate—an emulsifier and a thickening agent.

polyoxyethylene compounds—emulsifiers used in cosmetic formulations.

polyoxyethylene monooleate—an emulsifier. *See also* PEG 20-oleate.

polyoxyethylene nonylphenyl ether (AKA nonoxynol)—an emulsifier.

polyoxyethylene stearyl alcohol—an emulsifier. *See also* PEG stearol.

polyoxyethylene-(21)-steryl alcohol—an emulsifier. *See also* PEG-21 stearol.

polyoxyethyleneglycol monostearate—an emulsifier.

polypentaerythritol tetralaurate—an emulsifier. Considered a noncomedogenic raw material.

polypeptides—*see* hydrolyzed animal protein; protein.

polyphenol—the coloring agent in phenolic compounds. It is also considered a natural antiseptic. Polyphenol is rather irritating and sensitizing.

polyquaternium-10—a cellulose polymer and conditioning agent used in skin-conditioning formulations.

polyquaternium-24—suggested by some companies to be used as an SPF enhancer in sunscreen formulations. This is a film former similar to polyquaternium-10, but it gives better skin feel and has a lipophilic character that enables it to act as a secondary emulsifier and help form a thicker, more uniform sunscreen film.

polysaccharide xanthan—*see* xanthan gum.

polysorbate 20—a solubilizer, emulsifier, viscosity modifier, and stabilizer of essential oils in water.

polysorbate 40—an emulsifier and stabilizer of essential oils in water. It is also a detergent. Employed in a variety of cleansing and moisturizing preparations.

polysorbate 60—an emulsifier, wetting agent, and detergent emulsifier for mineral oil, fats, and waxes. It is also a stabilizer of essential oils in water. Widely used in cosmetic and toiletry preparations.

polysorbate 60 NF—an oil-in-water emulsifier and a fragrance solubilizer used in cosmetic and pharmaceutical creams and lotions. *See also* polysorbate 60.

polysorbate 80—an oil-in-water emulsifier.

polysorbate 80 NF—a hydrophilic emulsifier, pigment dispersant, and solubilizer for oils and fragrances. Used in creams, lotions, and makeup bases.

polysorbate 120—a fragrance solubilizer and an emulsifier used in sunscreen preparations and moisturizing creams and lotions.

polyvinyl acetate emulsion—a binder, emulsion stabilizer, and film-forming substance. *See also* polyvinylpyrrolidone.

polyvinyl alcohol—a binder, film former, and viscosity-increasing agent used primarily in makeup and nail polish preparations.

polyvinylpyrrolidone (AKA PVP)—perceivable benefits include water and wear resistance, pigment dispersion, a nongreasy feel, and improved stick integrity. PVPs are commonly found in waterproof sunscreens and mascaras and in lipsticks to improve their wear.

poplar bud extract—said to be antibactericidal and support wound healing. It may also be used topically for treating superficially broken skin as well as sunburn.

potassium PCA—a humectant that improves skin moisturizaion.

potassium alginate—*see* algin.

potassium alum (AKA alum)—a cosmetic astringent.

potassium carbomer 941—refer to carbomer entry in chapter 4.

potassium chloride—a laboratory reagent used as a viscosity-increasing agent in cosmetic and pharmaceutical preparations.

potassium hydroxide—used as an emulsifier in lotions and as an alkali in liquid soaps, protective creams, and shaving preparations. Depending on the concentration used, it can be highly irritating to the skin and/or cause a burning sensation.

potassium myristate—a cleansing and emulsifying agent.

potassium phosphate—a humectant and pH adjuster used in cosmetic formulations. Potassium phosphate is an inorganic salt.

potassium sorbate—a preservative primarily against mold and yeast and used in concentrations of 0.025–0.2%. It is nontoxic but may cause mild skin irritation.

potassium stearate—a cleansing and emulsifying agent.

potassium sulfate—a reagent in cosmetics. Potassium sulfate is an inorganic salt with a primary function as a viscosity-increasing agent.

PPG ceteareth 9—a surfactant and emulsifying agent.

PPG-5-ceteth 20—a surfactant and emulsifying agent.

PPG 30 cetyl ester—an emollient.

PPG 50 cetyl ester—an emollient.

PPG 2-PEG 20 isocetyl acetate—a fragrance solubilizer and oil-in-water emulsifier.

PPG-20 methyl glucose ether—an emollient.

PPG-4 myristyl ether propionate—an emollient.

pregnenolone hemisuccinate—used topically as an anti-inflammatory and anti-itch agent. A corticosteroid. See also primula extract.

primrose —see primula extract.

primula extract (*Primula officinalis* or *Primula vulagris*) (AKA primrose)—traditionally used as adjunct soothing and anti-itching treatment. It is useful in dry skin preparations. The leaves of some species are known to cause skin irritation sometimes resulting in a form of eczema.

procollagen—water-binding and moisturizing. Procollagen is a triple helical molecule of collagen and is fully soluble and membrane permeable. It is hygroscopic and, as such, is able to bind many times its weight in water. Procollagen is found naturally in the skin as a first stage in the production of collagen. With age, there is a decrease in the skin's procollagen content that may have some correlation to the increased dryness and reduction in elasticity often associated with mature skin.

proline—a skin-conditioning agent. An amino acid found in the collagen molecule. *See also* amino acid.

propanetriol—*see* glycerin.

propolis—once considered a mystical cure for such problems as infections and troubled skin. Chemists now recognize propolis as having a sun protective function, and many preparations for acne problems also contain propolis as an active substance for its healing and cleansing properties. Propolis is comprised of resins, balsam, various waxes, essential oils, pollen, flavonoids, amino acids, vitamins, and minerals. This is a component of beeswax, often referred to by beekeepers as "bee glue." It is collected from trees, shrubs, flowers, and other types of plants visited by bees.

propolis extract HD 10%—*see* propolis.

propyl gallate—an antioxidant with preservative properties.

propyl methoxycinnamate—a sunscreen chemical. *See also* methoxycinnamate.

propyl paraben—one of the most frequently used preservatives against bacteria and mold. It has a low sensitizing and low toxicity factor and is reputed to be very safe. Considered a noncomedogenic raw material.

propylene carbonate—used in chemical reactions as a solvent, plasticizer, solubilizer, or dilutent.

propylene glycol—next to water, this is the most common moisture-carrying vehicle used in cosmetic formulations. It has better skin permeation than glycerin, and it also gives a pleasant feel with less greasiness than glycerin. Propylene glycol is used as a humectant since it absorbs water from the air. It also serves as a solvent for antioxidants and preservatives. In addition, it has preservative properties against bacteria and fungi when used in concentrations of 16% or higher. There is a concern that propylene glycol is an irritant at high concentrations, though it appears to be quite safe at usage levels under 5%. *See also* glycerin.

propylene glycol ceteth-3 acetate—an emollient used in moisturizing preparations.

propylene glycol dicaprylate/dicaprate—has very good emollient properties. It also provides a product with good skin coverage and spreadability and absorption promotion properties. It does not cause skin irritation.

propylene glycol di-isostearate—considered an excellent emollient. Similar to jojoba oil.

propylene glycol di-pelargonate—an emollient ester with good skin-penetrating and spreadability properties. Does not leave a greasy feel.

propylene glycol mono-isostearate (AKA propylene glycol isostearate)—an emollient.

propylene glycol monomethyl ether—a stabilizer and skin penetration enhancer often found in topical acne preparations in which erythromycin is the active substance.

protein (AKA partially hydrolyzed protein; peptide; peptone; polypeptide)—its main function in skin care preparations is to produce a good film on the skin, thus helping reduce the loss of natural moisture. The films formed by animal proteins, such as collagen and elastin, are not occlusive as may be the case with mineral oil. Rather, they lie on the skin and have an affinity for it. All proteins, whether animal, vegetable, or silk derived, are built up from amino acids linked together to form a polymer. Depending on its source, the molecular weight of naturally occurring proteins may range from several thousands to millions, and the amino acid composition, which also influences the protein's properties, may vary widely. In the case of collagen-derived proteins, attributes include the ability to form clear solutions, contribute viscosity, stabilize oil-in-water emulsions, bind moisture, and form glossy films. The benefits claimed are a soft and silky skin feel, increased moisture retention with a related improvement of elasticity, and a decrease in chapping and irritation conditions. Adding protein to skin cleansing surfactants reduces skin irritation and dryness. Animal-derived collagen protein is still the preferred protein because of performance, ease of availability, and cost. However, due to consumer preferences to move away from animal products, vegetal proteins are being perfected for use in skin care cosmetics. The most popular appears to be wheat-based hydrolyzed protein. Proteins are usually hydrolyzed to achieve lower molecular values, which enhances moisture-binding properties.

pseudocollagen—acts in much the same way as collagen, leaving the skin feeling soft and supple. Pseudocollagen forms a moisture retentive film on the skin in a similar way to soluble collagen. It represents the pseudocollagenous extract of yeast cells. It is plant derived.

pumice powder—usually employed in cosmetics for removing tough or rough skin. Used in hand cleansing preparations, skin cleansing grains, powders, and soaps for acne. Because of its abrasive action, daily use is not recommended. If used continuously on dry, sensitive skin, it will most likely cause irritation. It can also be an irritant when used in soapless detergents. Pumice is of volcanic origin and consists primarily of complex silicates of aluminum and alkali metals.

purcellin oil (nonanimal) (AKA cetearyl octanoate)—used as a fixative in perfumes. This is a synthetic mixture of fatty esters designed to simulate the natural oil obtained from the preen glands of waterfowl.

PVP—*see* polyvinylpyrrolidone.

PVP/eicosene copolymer—a waterproofing polymer with sunscreen absorption properties. *See also* polyvinylpyrrolidone.

PVP/hexdecene copolymer—designed for use in formulations where unique delivery systems are desired. *See also* polyvinylpyrrolidone.

PVP/triacontene copolymer—one of the newest PVPs. It has a greater waterproofing effect and significantly improved retention of UV absorbers in sunscreen products than PVP/eicosene. *See also* polyvinylpyrrolidone.

pyridoxine dipalmitate—a skin-conditioning agent used in moisturizing formulations.

pyridoxine tripalmitate—soothing to the skin. This is a stable, oil-soluble form of vitamin B_6. It prevents scaling and skin dryness and is also used as a product texturizer.

pyrodixine hydrochloride—a skin-conditioning agent that is also widely used in hair products.

pyrodoxine HCL—*see* pyrodixine hydrochloride.

L-pyroglutaminic acid—*see* PCA.

pyrrolidonic carbon acid (AKA nalidone)—a natural moisturizing factor that protects the skin from dehydration and increases its moisture-retention capabilities.

pyrrolidone-carboxylic acid—a moisturizing agent. *See also* PCA.

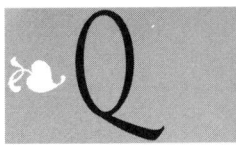

quassia *(Picraena excelsa)*—an antibacterial. Quassia yields quassin, a bitter alkaloid obtained from the wood of *Quassia amara*. Quassia is primarily a denaturant for ethyl alcohol.

quaternium 15—an all-purpose preservative active against bacteria, mold, and yeast and used in concentrations of 0.02–0.3%. Though not a primary skin irritant, quaternium 15 is considered a highly sensitizing preservative when used in leave-on cosmetic preparations. Dermatologists find it to be the most frequent sensitizer among preservatives in the United States. It is probably the greatest formaldehyde releaser among cosmetic preservatives, causing dermatitis in people allergic to formaldehyde and even to those who are not. The technical data of some manufacturers indicates, however, that quaternium-15 does not contain or release free gaseous formaldehyde. These would most likely be versions of quaternium-15 that have been specially formulated and adjusted to avoid formaldehyde release.

quaternium 18—*see* quaternium 15.

quaternium 18 hectorite—used as a thickener and suspending agent. Produced by a reaction of hectorite and the quaternary salt. Used in concentrations of 1.5%. *See also* hectorite; quaternium 15.

quercus extract (AKA English oak extract)—*see* oak.

quinaquina —*see* cinchona extract.

quince extract *(Pyrus cydonia)*—mentioned as appropriate for use in cosmetics for dry skin and eye treatment preparations. *See also* quince seed.

quince seed—an emollient, emulsifier, and thickening agent. Obtained from the dried seeds of *Cydonia oblonga*. It may cause allergic reactions.

quinine extract—an alkaloid from the bark of *Cinchona officinalis*. *See also* cinchona extract.

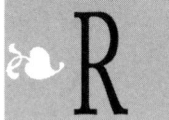

raspberry concentrate *(Rubus idaeus)*—botanical properties are described as astringent and tonic. Raspberry concentrate is added to cosmetics to give them the fruit's fresh smell. Some sources claim that there is no evidence of raspberries having any external value for the skin, and they may increase allergenicity.

red algae extracts—*see* seaweed extract.

red clover—described as beneficial for acne and eczema. *See also* clover.

red petrolatum—one of the 21 FDA-approved sunscreen chemicals with an approved usage level of 30–100%. Not commonly used.

red poppy extract *(Papaver rhoeas)*—considered a soothing emollient.

red raspberry extract—considered astringent. *See also* raspberry concentrate.

red vine extract—anti-inflammatory and anti-itching. Traditionally used upon manifestation of broken or fragile capillaries.

red wine—contains tartaric acid, a member of the alpha hydroxyacid family. *See also* alpha hydroxyacid.

resin—used to give gloss, flow, adhesion, and water resistance to cosmetics. This is a brittle substance, usually translucent or transparent, that can be either naturally derived or synthetically obtained. Among the natural resins are dammar, elemi, and sandarac, formed from the hardened secretions of these plants. Toxicity and allergenicity depend upon ingredients used.

resorcinol—in very mild solutions it is used as an antiseptic and as a soothing preparation for itchy skin. In slightly higher concentrations it removes the surface layer of skin (the dry, dead cells) and is used in lotions for irritated skin and particularly in connection with acne. In still higher concentrations it can act as an aggressive surface skin exfoliant. Resorcinol can also be used as a preservative. While it is a beneficial skin care ingredient when used in low concentrations, it causes irritation in higher concentrations, with a strong burning sensation and a reddening of the skin. Used in high concentrations as a peel, resorcinol may cause a variety of problems, including swelling. Resorcinol is obtained from various resins.

restharrow extract *(Ononis arvensis* and *Ononis spinosa)*—an emollient that provides relief for skin itching. Traditionally used for relieving the problems of eczema. The extract is obtained from the plant's roots.

reticulin (soluble)—a protein that, when on the skin's surface, acts as a protective agent against water loss. It helps increase the water content of the skin's outer layers, plumping up the epidermis and leaving the skin softer and smoother. Unlike proteins of a similar molecular weight, when reticulin dries it leaves the skin feeling pleasant and without tackiness.

retinol—considered a skin revitalizer.

retinol trilinolein—probably a free radical scavenger.

retinyl palmitate (AKA vitamin A palmitate)—a skin-conditioning agent. The ester of retinol and palmitic acid. *See also* vitamin A palmitate.

retinyl palmitate polypeptide—allows for the delivery of vitamin A as a water dispersable substance.

riboflavin (AKA Vitamin B_2)—used in skin care preparations as an emollient. Medicinally, it is used for the treatment of skin lesions.

riboflavin tetraacetate—a skin-conditioning agent. A vitamin B_2 derivative. *See also* vitamin B.

ribonucleic acid (AKA RNA)—a surface film-forming agent with moisturizing action. This is the polyribonucleotide found in both the nucleus and the cytoplasm of cells.

rice flour—*see* rice starch.

rice oil *(Oryza sativa)*—recommended for combination skin products where the ingredients must not be too aggressive for the dry skin area and yet should be helpful for the oily T-zone.

rice bran extract—soothing. Recommended for treatment of dry, mature skin.

rice bran oil—a carrier and a soothing emollient. The germ and bran of unpolished rice contains linolic acid or vitamin F, oleic acid, palmitic acid, vitamin E, and oryzanol. The oil is expressed from rice bran.

rice germ oil—*see* rice bran oil.

rice starch—a demulcent and emollient. It forms a soothing, protective film when applied and is used in baby and face powders. Rice starch is a crystalline polymeric compound obtained from grains of rice.

ricinoleamide DEA—an emulsifier with lubricity and good wetting and softening properties. It can also serve as a foam booster and formula stabilizer when blended with anionic surfactants such as lauryl sulfates.

ricinoleth 40 (AKA PEG 40 ricinoleyl ether)—a surfactant used as a cleansing and solubilizing agent.

RNA—*see* ribonucleic acid.

roe extract *(Acipenser stellatus)* (AKA caviar)—used in products for oily and mature dehydrated skins in need for revitalization. It has a high- and wide-ranging vitamin content that includes vitamins A, D, E, B_1, B_2, and B_6. Roe extract contains an array of other constituents including cobalt, copper, fluorine, iodine, iron, magnesium, manganese, phosphorus, silicium, and zinc. The amino acids present are glutamic acid, glycine, methionine, lysine, arginine, histidine, and aspartic acid. In addition, roe has essential and sulfured amino acids and unsaturated fatty acids. Usage levels range from 1–5% depending on the preparation. Prepared from sturgeon roe.

Roman chamomile oil *(Anthemis nobilis)*—the most popular variety of chamomile. Different from German chamomile (AKA matricaria). Considered tonic and healing. *See also* chamomile.

rose extract *(Rosa* sp.)—credited with astringent, tonic, and deodorant properties. It is also used as a fragrance.

rose hips—a rose extract rich in vitamin C. *See also* vitamin C.

rose hips oil—described as a healing oil due to its antiseptic properties. It may also help regulate oil gland secretion. *See also* rose hips.

rose hips powder—*see* rose hips.

rose oil—has been credited with antiseptic, disinfectant, slightly tonic, and soothing properties. Some sources also cite moisturizing and moisture-retention abilities. It is found helpful in cases of skin redness or inflammation and where moisturization and regeneration is needed. Rose oil may be beneficial to all skin types particularly mature, dry, or sensitive skins. As real rose oil is only used in very high-grade perfumes, it is rosewater that is widely used in cosmetics and perfumery. As one of the most expensive essential oils, rose oil is almost always adulterated with substances like geranium, lemongrass, palmarosa, and terpene alcohols. The process of adulteration has become so refined that it is almost impossible to discover frauds. To produce rose oil, rose buds are picked for only a few hours in the morning, right after the dew, and are immediately distilled. According to some sources, 30 roses are required to make 1 drop of oil. It is considered the least toxic of all essences.

rose petal extract—has mild astringency and tonic value. *See also* rose extract.

rose wax—floral waxes, such as rose, jasmine, and others, complement the skin's natural lipids and give a product wear- and smudge-resistant properties. Rose wax is an almost odorless residue left after the extraction of the oily fractions.

rosemary extract *(Rosmarinus officinalis)*—a general effect attributed to this herb is the promotion of wound healing. It is also said to have astringent, toning, stimulating, deodorant, antiseptic, reactivating, antibacterial, softening, and invigorating properties. It also helps improve blood circulation thereby aiding in skin regeneration. Rosemary adds fragrance to a formulation. According to some sources, rosemary has antioxidant properties, making it effective for antiaging products. Some constituents of rosemary extract include a variety of amino acids, caffaic acid, rosemary acid, and apigenin. The leaf is the part of the plant used.

rosemary oil—credited with antiseptic properties. It is considered beneficial for acne, dermatitis, and eczema. Some reports indicate that rosemary oil may stimulate fibroblast growth with a possible increase in epidermal cell turnover. This would make it useful in products for aging and aged skin. Rosemary oil, obtained through distillation of the herb's flowering tops, is superior to that which is obtained via distillation of the stems and leaves. The latter process, however, is more common among the commercial oils.

rosewater—credited with soothing, astringent, and cleansing properties. In addition, it can be used as a vehicle for other ingredients and as an eye lotion. Ointment of rosewater is said to have soothing and cooling properties when applied to abrasions and other superficial skin lesions. Rosewater is often mixed with glycerin, which provides moisturization and lubricity. *See also* rose oil.

rosewax—*see* rose wax.

rosewood oil—one of the major perfumery oils used as a middle note. Until recently it was little used in aromatherapy. Although it does not have major curative power, rosewood oil appears useful as a cellular stimulant and tissue regenerator. As such it would be applicable to sensitive and aged skin, wrinkles, and general skin care. It is very mild and safe to use and is obtained via distillation of the chopped wood.

royal jelly—some sources claim that when used in cosmetic preparations, it favors the regeneration of dermal tissue. Other sources indicate that its use for topical cosmetic application has no proven cosmetic value. Royal jelly is produced by bees (for the nutrition of the queen bee) and is a mixture of proteins, fats, carbohydrates, water, growth factors, and various trace elements.

royal jelly extract HD—an extract of royal jelly. *See also* royal jelly.

Russian white oil—*see* mineral oil.

rutin—described as having tightening and strengthening properties for skin capillaries, thus helping to prevent a couperose condition. Rutin is found in rue leaves, buckwheat, and other plants.

rutine salt—*see* rutin.

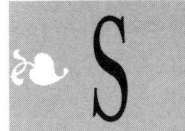

sacred bark—*see* cascara sagrada extract.

safflower oil *(Carthamus tinctorius)*—a carrier oil also considered hydrating to the skin. It consists primarily of linoleic acid triglycerides. Safflower oil is a noncomedogenic raw material obtained from the plant's seeds.

sage extract *(Salvia officinalis)*—considered to have astringent, antibacterial, antiseptic, anti-inflammatory, stimulating, softening, invigorating, and healing properties. Sage extract was traditionally used as a remedy for every type of inflammation. The extract is obtained from the herb's leaves.

sage oil—credited with depurative and healing properties and indicated for acne and oily skin. Sage oil is obtained by distillation of sage leaves and flowers. *See also* sage extract.

St. John's wort extract *(Hypericum perforatum)* (AKA hypericum extract)—said to have astringent, anti-inflammatory, and possibly soothing properties. St. John's wort offers general skin protection especially for sensitive skin and areas with burns. This is an herbaceous perennial plant with hypericine as its important constituent.

St. John's wort oil—considered anti-inflammatory. It is beneficial for sensitive and/or rough, chapped skin as well as acne skin or skin suffering from irritation and inflammation. It is also considered effective for improving capillary circulation. In addition, St. John's wort oil is an antibiotic and therefore a natural preservative. This is a deep red oil. *See also* St. John's wort extract.

salicylamide—an analgesic, fungicide, and anti-inflammatory ingredient used to soothe the skin. Salicylamide is an aromatic amide.

salicylic acid—has keratolytic activity when used in proper concentrations. It helps dissolve the top layer of corneum cells and improves the look and feel of the skin. Salicylic acid is also an antiseptic. Some sources report that it enhances the activity of other preservatives. Though it is widely used in acne soaps and lotions, some of its derivatives, such as 5-octanoylsalicylic acid, are being used for the treatment of aging skin. Salicylic acid can be absorbed through the skin and may cause skin redness and rashes, especially at high concentrations. Salicylic acid is a chemical found in some plants, particularly the leaves of wintergreen and the bark of sweet birch.

salt—*see* sodium chloride.

sambucus extract—*see* elder extract.

sandalwood oil *(Santalum album)* (AKA santal; santalum)—credited with astringent, anti-inflammatory, antibacterial, tonic, and soothing properties. It is also considered a good antiseptic in cases of acne and an astringent for oily skin. There are indications that sandalwood oil may promote epidermal cell turnover as some report it may stimulate growth of fibroblast. In addition, some manufacturers utilize it as a natural colorant to give products a light red or rose tone. Sandalwood oil may produce a rash in hypersensitive people, especially if it is present in high concentrations. Produced by distillation of the inner wood.

santal oil—*see* sandalwood oil.

santalum oil—*see* sandalwood oil.

saponaria extract—*see* soapwort extract.

sarriette oil—a fragrance with healing, tonic, and anti-inflammatory properties.

sarsasparilla *(Smilax officinalis)*—therapeutic botanical claims for skin problems include healing, antiseptic, and beneficial for chronic skin disease. Independent of the variety, in every case the sarsasparilla's root is the part used.

sassafras oil *(Sassafras albidum)*—credited with antiseptic, astringent, and stimulant properties. Its main active ingredient is saprol, constituting about 80%. Sassafras oil is obtained from the plant's bark and root through a process of steam distillation. It may produce dermatitis in hypersensitive individuals.

savory *(Satureia hortensis)* (AKA hortrensis extract)—considered antiseptic and antibiotic. It is indicated for acne skin. A hardy herb.

scabwort—*see* elecampane.

sclary sage oil—*see* clary sage oil.

scurvy grass extract *(Cochlearia officinalis)*—considered tonic. It is a source of vitamin C.

SD alcohol 40—*see* alcohol SD-40.

SD alcohol 40A—*see* alcohol SDA-40.

sea clay—*see* clay.

sea minerals yeast derivative—described as supplying "essential minerals" for cosmetic applications. Marine elements have been used since time immemorial for their beneficial effects on all epidermal structures. The mixture of sea elements with low-molecular-weight yeast glycoproteins apparently results in a degree of biocompatability with the skin and acceptance by the epidermal cells.

sea salt—a mild abrasive used in scrubs. Its water solubility allows it to self-dissolve during product use. It is also employed as a dilutant. As sea salt does not seem to form secondary reactions, it is considered a stable ingredient in cosmetic formulations. In large grains, it is colored and perfumed and utilized in bath salts. Sea salt may cause dryness.

sea wave—*see* seaweed extract.

sea wrack—*see* seaweed extract.

seawater—healing powers have long been attributed to the sea. Salt water can have an antiseptic, debriding, or stimulating effect when used to treat wounds. However, oligotherapy, also referred to as thalassatherapy, has yet to demonstrate a truly positive effect on cosmetic properties of the skin.

seaweed (fresh)—has gelatinous properties. It is the major ingredient in the thin, clear masks, that peel off in one piece when applied on the skin. This type of mask allows the skin to build up a supply of water and gives it a moist, supple look. Seaweed is also used in face creams and lotions, providing body and substance to products. Considered good for oily skin.

seaweed extract *(Fucus vesiculosus)* (AKA algae extract; black tang; bladderwrack; fucus; kelp; sea wave; seawrack)— Seaweed has been used by the Chinese for curing burns and rashes; by the Polynesians for treating wounds, bruises, and swelling; and by mariners who recognized its healing properties. Seaweed is found to be stimulating, revitalizing, and nourishing to the skin due to its iodine and sulfur amino acid content, which also give it anti-inflammatory and disinfectant abilities. Seaweed's moisturizing properties are attributed to its ability to react with protein and form a protective gel on the skin's surface, reducing moisture loss due to evaporation. It has potential tissue renewal action and positive effects on facial wrinkles probably because of its silicon content. It protects sensitive skin against irritation, making it particularly effective in shaving creams. It is also beneficial for treating mature and drier skins due to its smoothing and softening actions. Seaweed extract seems to be effective in treating acne based on its presumed antibiotic properties, which offer the skin protection against infection. Evidence indicates seaweed may help accelerate wound healing and improve the healing of burns (including sunburns) and other wounds when in the presence of calcium alginate. It can be utilized as a regenerator in cases of suntanned or "orange peeled" skin. It reportedly improves blood circulation in the skin. Due to its alginates, seaweed is also used by formulators as a thickener for gellants and emulsions. In cosmetic products its total percentage of use varies between 2% and 7%. The benefits of seaweed and seaweed extracts can be attributed to the plants wealth of components that include water, mineral matters, lipids, protids, glucids, and sulfuric esters. Its vitamin content includes vitamins A, B_1, B_2, B_3, B_5, B_{12}, C, D, E, and K. Among its mineral constituents are iodine, calcium, iron, phosphorus, sodium, potassium, zinc, nitrogen, copper, chlorine, magnesium, and manganese. It has trace amounts of various other minerals such as silver, lithium, silicon, bromine, titanium, cobalt, and arsenic. The amino acid content of seaweed is extremely high compared to other plants, and its polysaccharides include fructose, galactose, glucose, mannose, and xylose. Additional constituents include folic acid, choline, alginic acid, uronic acid, alginates, carrageenan, cellulose, proteins, agar-agar, algin, and iodine-protein complexes. There are more than 17,000 seaweed species that are classified according to color—green, blue, red, and brown. The red and brown varieties, the most commonly used in cosmetic preparations and generally referred to as seaweed or algae extract, are green when fresh and olive-brown when dry. The thallus is the part used for cosmetic purposes.

selenium—used for years in topical preparations for its antifungal properties. Selenium has been shown to have other protective effects such as repairing DNA, reducing the DNA-binding of carcinogens, and suppressing gene mutations. In laboratory studies, skin lotions containing selenium compounds have been shown to decrease skin damage induced by UV irradiation such as inflammation, blistering, and pigmentation.

serine—a hydrophilic amino acid. Serine helps retain the skin's moisture balance. *See also* amino acid; protein.

serum albumen (AKA serum algumin)—bovine serum albumen is a good carrier of essential fatty acids to epidermal cells. When applied to the skin in combination with essential fatty acids, it is said to help increase the rate of epidermal cell renewal. Serum albumen is the fluid remaining after the removal of fibrin clot and blood cells.

serum algumin—*see* serum albumen.

serum protein—contains all essential amino acids. By varying the process it is possible to concentrate fractions that have high specific essential amino acid contents, such as methionine and lysine. Made by a selected fractionation process to isolate the plasma serum proteins present. *See also* amino acid; protein.

sesame oil—a commonly used carrier oil for cosmetic products, it has the same emollient properties as other nut and vegetable oils. Sesame oil is useful in suntan lotions as it

Gene

WHILE YOU WERE OUT

Tamara

Phone Numbers

ice		
Area Code	Number	Ext.
icemail		
X		
ger		
obile		
mail		

☐ Telephoned
☐ Please call
☐ Returned your call
☐ Called to see you
☐ Wants to see you
☐ Will call again
☐ URGENT

Message

Sunscreen in Graham Web
s shay butter

Operator

blocks 30% of the sun's burning UV rays. Derived from sesame seeds.

shaddock extract—an extract obtained from the fruit of *Citrus grandis*. It is an unusual pear-shaped citrus fruit similar to a grapefruit.

shave grass—*see* horsetail extract.

shea butter—protects the skin from dehydration and other climatic influences. It is a natural fat obtained from the fruit of the karite tree.

shea butter (hydrodispersible)—an excellent emollient for use in creams, lotions, and makeup preparations. It alleviates skin dryness and has sun-protection and high skin-penetration properties. Obtained by the hydroxylation of shea butter.

shinleaf extract *(Pyrola elliptica)*—a botanical reported to help maintain the balance of normal skin.

silica—a carrier for emollients. It is also used in sunscreens. Spherical silica is porous and highly absorbent, with absorption capabilities being roughly 1.5 times its weight. A typical claim associated with silica is oil control. Tests show it has been successfully used in hypoallergenic and allergy tested formulations.

silicon glyconucleopeptides—a conditioning agent. This is protein attached to a silicone.

silicon oil—a generic description usually referring to dimethicone.

silicone (volatile)—used in face creams to increase the product's protection capabilities against water evaporation from the skin. Silicone polyethers are mainly used in water-based skin care formulations and give improved softness, gloss, and feel. Silicones have been used in cosmetics for more than 30 years. As they are minerals able to repel water, silicones present formulation problems because of poor compatibility with cosmetic oils and emollients. Silicones are not irritating.

silicone wax—gives the formulation improved glide on the skin.

silicum—used in scrubbing preparations for its roughness and texture.

silk amino acids—a silk-derived protein resulting from the complete hydrolysis of silk. *See also* amino acids; silk protein.

silk powder—recommended primarily for use in powder make-ups to improve humectancy, oil absorption, and anti-cracking properties. However, a large amount of silk powder may be needed to obtain the desired results. Silk powder is a micronized powder of natural silk fibroin and is not compatible with all inorganic pigments used in color cosmetics. Obtained from the secretion of the silkworm. Silk powder may cause allergic skin reactions.

silk proteins—protect the skin from dehydration and leave it with a smooth feel. Described as very effective for use in eye wrinkle creams. It is being claimed that their low molecular weight allows for penetration in the top layers of the corneum layer.

silverweed—*see* cinquefoil extract.

slippery elm extract *(Ulmus fulva)*—said to be soothing and emollient. It is found to be beneficial in aftershave preparations and for treating sunburn. *See also* slippery elm bark extract.

slippery elm bark extract—considered to have soothing, antiseptic, anti-inflammatory, and healing action. The inner bark is considered to have important medicinal value. Microscopic examination of the bark's tissue shows round starch grains and very characteristic twin crystals of calcium oxalate.

soap bark—a natural surfactant used for its cleansing properties. Some sources indicate a high allergenicity potential.

soapwort extract *(Saponaria officinalis)*—Credited with cleansing properties due to its saponin content. It is also said to be soothing to the skin and relieve itching. The extract is made primarily from the roots of this herbaceous perennial.

sodium alginate—*see* algin.

SOD—*see* superoxide dimutase.

sodium aluminosilicate—*see* sodium aluminum silicate.

sodium aluminum chlorohydroxy lactate — a cosmetic astringent. This is an inorganic salt.

sodium aluminum silicate (AKA sodium aluminosilicate; sodium silicoaluminate)—abrasive. It is a viscosity-increasing agent.

sodium benzoate—a nontoxic, organic salt preservative particularly effective against yeast, with some activity against molds and bacteria. Generally used in concentrations of 0.1–0.2%.

sodium bicarbonate (AKA baking soda)—an inorganic salt used as a buffering agent and a pH adjuster. Used in skin-smoothing powders. It also serves as a neutralizer.

sodium bisulfate—an inorganic salt used as an antiseptic and a pH adjuster in cosmetic creams. Concentrated solutions can produce strong irritation.

sodium bisulfite—a preservative and antioxidant.

sodium borate—a preservative and emulsifier with astringent and antiseptic properties. It is also used as a pH adjuster. Sodium borate is the sodium salt of boric acid. It may cause skin dryness and irritation.

sodium cetearyl sulfate—a surfactant used as a cleansing agent. Also an oil-in-water emulsifier for creams.

sodium chloride (AKA table salt)—used as a preservative, astringent, and antiseptic to treat inflamed lesions. Diluted solutions are not considered irritating.

sodium chondroitin sulfate—described as a skin conditioning agent for use in moisturizers and night skin care preparations. A derivative of a natural mucopolysaccharide. *See also* mucopolysaccharides.

sodium citrate—may be used to bind (via a chelating action) trace metals in solutions and as an alkalizer in cosmetic formulations. It is the sodium salt of citric acid.

sodium cocoate—a surfactant used as an emulsifying and cleansing agent primarily in bath soaps and cleansers. This sodium salt of coconut acid may also be listed as coconut oil. *See also* coconut oil.

sodium coco hydrolyzed collagen—a surfactant that is non-irritating to the skin or mucous membranes.

sodium cocoyl isethionate—a mild, high-foaming surfactant. Leaves the skin with a soft afterfeel.

sodium cocoylsarcosinate—a surfactant used as a cleansing agent.

sodium dehydroacetate—a preservative against bacteria and fungi that is used at concentration levels of 1.0% or less.

It is useful in combination with parabens. May cause skin irritation.

sodium dihydroxycetyl phosphate—a surfactant used as a cleansing agent.

sodium hexametaphosphate—a chelating agent and a corrosion inhibitor. This is an inorganic salt.

sodium hyaluronate—used as a moisturizing agent, viscosifier, and emulsifier, sodium hyaluronate is capable of binding 1,800 times its own weight in water. It is the sodium salt of hyaluronic acid. *See also* hyaluronic acid.

sodium hydroxide—commonly referred to as caustic soda. It is a chemical reagent used in making soap. If too concentrated it may cause severe skin irritation.

sodium lactate—keeps a product's pH from becoming too acidic. Sodium lactate is naturally occurring on skin and is moisturizing and moisture-binding. It is also used as a substitute for glycerin.

sodium lactate methylsilanol—an additive used in self-tanning preparations. It helps in obtaining a more uniform color.

sodium laureth-5 carboxylate—a very mild surfactant. It substantially improves the skin's tolerance to cleansers. It also has good emulsifying properties and is insensitive to water hardness.

sodium laureth-11 carboxylate—a surfactant. *See also* sodium laureth-5 carboxylate; sodium laureth-13 carboxylate.

sodium laureth-13 carboxylate—an extremely mild surfactant that substantially improves the skin's tolerance of cleansers. It is particularly suitable for high-quality formulations, baby shampoos, and products designed for sensitive skin. This ingredient has good emulsifying properties and is insensitive to water hardness.

sodium laureth sulfate—a versatile surfactant used in personal care products. It enjoys good skin compatibility and is very often found in shower foams, foam bath products, and liquid soaps. It exhibits a moderate skin irritation index in irritation tests.

sodium lauroamphoacetate—a mild surfactant that is especially suitable for use in products where skin tolerance is important (e.g., baby and child care products).

sodium lauryl sarcosinate—a foaming agent used primarily in hair products.

sodium lauryl sulfate—serves as a base surfactant, foaming agent with good foaming properties, dispersant, and wetting agent. Formulators have found it ideal for cleansers and soaps intended to be packaged with pump dispensers. It is found to be moderately to significantly irritating.

sodium magnesium silicate—a binder and bulking agent used primarily in makeup products.

sodium mannuronate methylsilanol—a skin-conditioning agent.

sodium methylcocoyl taurate—an emulsifier and mild cleansing agent. Used in cleansing creams, lotions, shampoos, and bath soaps. Derived from coconut oil.

sodium methyloleoyl taurate—an emulsifier and a mild cleansing and foaming agent derived from oleic acid.

sodium oleate—a mild cleansing and foaming agent generally used in soaps. Derived from natural fats and oils.

sodium PCA (AKA Ajidew NaPCA)—a high-performance humectant due to its moisture-binding ability. It is derived from amino acids. Sodium PCA also exists naturally in the skin as a component of the natural moisturizing factor. It is considered a noncomedogenic, nonallergenic raw material recommended for dry, delicate, and sensitive skins.

sodium PCS (AKA Ajidew N-50)—a humectant. *See also* PCA; sodium PCA.

sodium phosphate—helps maintain product pH.

sodium polyacrylate—a suspending agent, stabilizer, and emulsifier.

sodium polyacrylate starch—a thickener and gellant with good pH stability.

sodium polyphosphate—a preservative against bacteria, molds, and yeasts. Used at high concentrations, it can cause skin irritation.

sodium polystyrene sulfonate—a film former. It holds the actives on site and gives the feeling of skin tightening. Obtained from synthetic sources.

sodium ricinolate—an emulsifying agent used in certain soaps and medicines. It is a sodium salt of the fatty acids from castor oil.

sodium silicoaluminate—*see* sodium aluminum silicate.

sodium stearate—a fatty acid used as a waterproofing agent. One of the least allergy-causing sodium salts of fatty acids. Nonirritating to the skin. *See also* stearic acid.

sodium sulfate—a filler in the manufacturing of synthetic detergents and soaps. A laboratory reagent. It may enhance the irritant action of certain detergents.

sodium sulfite—has antiseptic, preservative, and antioxidant properties. Sodium sulfite is also a topical antifungal.

sodium tallowate (AKA tallow)—a defoamer, emollient, intermediate, and surface active agent. *See also* tallow.

sodium/TEA lauryl—a moderately irritating surfactant.

sodium tetraborate—*see* sodium borate.

sodium triceth sulfate—a surfactant.

sodium trideceth sulfate—a surfactant used as a cleansing and emulsifying agent. Its activity and level of irritation depends on the formulation's pH.

soluble elastin—*see* tropoelastin.

sorbic acid—a broad-spectrum, nontoxic preservative against molds and yeasts with moderate sensitizing potential in leave-on cosmetics. It is used in concentrations of 0.1–0.3%, and its activity is dependant on the formulation's pH. Sorbic acid is used as a replacement for glycerin in emulsions, ointments, and various cosmetic creams. Obtained from the berries of the mountain ash. It can also be produced synthetically. Sorbic acid can be irritating.

sorbitan isostearate—an emulsifier used in the preparation of sunscreens, moisturizing creams, and lotions.

sorbitan laurate—an emulsifier in cosmetic creams and lotions as well as a stabilizer of essential oils in water.

sorbitan monostearate—*see* sorbitan stearate.

sorbitan oleate—a mild emulsifier derived from sugar.

sorbitan palmitate—an emulsifier with moisture-binding abilities. It also serves as a solubilizer of essential oils in water. Derived from sorbitol.

sorbitan sesquioleate—a surfactant used as an emulsifying agent. *See also* sorbitol.

sorbitan stearate—an emulsifier for water-in-oil creams and lotions and a solubilizer of essential oils in water. It results from the reaction of stearic acid with sorbitol and is therefore synthetically produced from naturally derived materials.

sorbitan trioleate—an emulsifier. *See also* sorbitol.

sorbitan tristearate—an emulsifier and alternate for sorbitan stearate.

sorbitate stearate—a secondary emulsifier that helps formulate glossy emulsions.

sorbitol—absorbs moisture from the air to prevent skin dryness and leaves the skin feeling smooth and velvety. However, if the skin's moisture content is greater than that of the atmosphere, it will draw moisture out of the skin, thereby increasing the feeling of dryness. Sorbitol is used by formulators as a replacement for glycerin in emulsions, ointments, and various cosmetic creams. Obtained from the leaves and in some cases the berries of mountain ash. Sorbitol also occurs in other berries (except grapes), cherries, plums, pears, apples, seaweed, and algae.

sorrel extract *(Rumex acetosa)*—an astringent. Though there are many varieties of sorrel, including wood sorrel, French sorrel, and garden sorrel, similar properties are attributed to all. The extract is obtained from the whole herb or just from the leaves.

southernwood extract *(Artemisia abrotanum)*—botanical sources cite it as having antiseptic and tonic properties. The extract is obtained from the whole plant.

soy bean oil (AKA soybean oil)—often used as a smoothing ingredient. It has a high content of phosphatides (e.g., lecithin), sterols, and vitamins (A, E, and K). It is reportedly used in numerous forms, including hydrogenated, maleated, and unsaponified. Considered by some sources to be somewhat comedogenic, soy bean oil is not irritating.

soy bean oil (unsaponified)—possibly has a similar action to true biological precursors. It has a small molecular structure and is thought to act more as a hormonelike cellular messenger once it reaches the epidermal keratinocytes and, particularly, the dermal fibroblast. It is said to stimulate the synthesis of collagen, elastin, proteoglycans, and structural glycoproteins.

soy germ oil—*see* soy bean oil.

soy oil—*see* soy bean oil.

soy amino acids—*see* amino acid.

soy lecithin—a mild refattening agent that can be effectively used in facial cleansers formulated for dry skin.

soy sterol—an emulsifier, emollient, and emulsion stabilizer. Soy sterol is considered a noncomedogenic raw material.

soybean oil—*see* soy bean oil.

spearmint oil *(Mentha viridis)*—a cooling, aromatic stimulant described as having cleansing and decongesting properties. Indicated for acne and oily skin. Its fragrance and therapeutic activity is similar to that of peppermint but fresher and less harsh. *See also* mint oil.

spermaceti—a waxy substance used in the manufacture of cosmetics to thicken the products and give them shine. Originally obtained from whales as a source of fish oil, it is now synthetic. Spermaceti is nontoxic and nonirritating.

sphingolipids—one of the newest ingredients available. Sphingolipids are ceramide precursors with unique moisturizing properties. They appear to work with the cellular system in providing a restorative effect on a damaged or disturbed corneum layer. Researchers are speculating that sphingolipids may also exhibit cell-regulating functions. Sphingolipids have been found in various mammalian cell types with higher concentrations present in the brain and spinal cord. Although individual plants contain sphingolipids, the quantities of available sphingolipids are too small to isolate in an efficient and economical manner. The synthesized version does not exhibit exactly the same properties as the natural one. The use of sphingolipids in cosmetics is limited by availability and price. Sphingolipid liposomes are called sphingosomes.

sphinogoceryl—forms a protective film that strengthens the skin's ability to protect against toxins and increases the skin's moisture-retention abilities. It can also improve skin texture.

sphingomyelin—can be used as an amphiphilic liposome component in the manufacture of the liposome capsule.

sphingomyelinase—a fluid that can enhance the skin's moisture-retention properties.

spinal cord ox-beef purified extracts—*see* hydrolyzed animal protein.

***Spiraea* extract**—*see* meadowsweet.

spirulina extract—said to have a hydrating effect on the skin's surface layers. Botanical claims also maintain that certain spirulina proteins contribute to the stimulation of the fibroblast and to tissue regeneration.

spruce oil *(Picea excelsa)*—like sandalwood, rosemary, and jasmine oils, spruce oil has been observed to stimulate fibroblast growth. While the relevance of this observation has not been scientifically established, it has been noticed that stimulation of fibroblast activity could result in an increase in epidermal cell turnover. Spruce oil is produced by distillation of spruce branches.

squalane (AKA squalene)—an excellent moisturizer and lubricant. Its compatibility with skin lipids can be attributed to the fact that human sebum is comprised of 25% squalane. Squalane is obtained by hydrogenation of shark liver oil or other natural oils. Components found in fish oils may reduce skin irritation and allergic responses. It can also be obtained from plant sources.

squalane and squalene and glycolipids and phytosterols and tocopharol—a light emollient that contains natural lipids also found in the skin. This is a natural plant cell oil extract, not a mixture as the name suggests.

squalene—*see* squalane.

starch gum—*see* dextrin.

stearalkonium hectorite—*see* hectorite.

stearamide DEA (AKA stearic acid diethanolamide)—a thickener and a wax emulsifier used in soaps, creams, and lotions.

stearamidopropyl dimethylamine—a surfactant and conditioner for mild facial cleansers, mild hand cleansers, and baby products. It is very mild to the skin and eyes.

stearate—*see* sodium stearate.

stearate SE—*see* sodium stearate.

steareth-2—an emulsifier for oil-in-water systems. This is a polyoxyethylene ether of fatty alcohol.

steareth-7—an emulsifier for oil-in-water formulations.

steareth-10—an emulsifier for oil-in-water formulations particularly creams and lotions of high stability. Some sources indicate it as having a comedogenicity and moderate irritancy potential.

steareth-20—an emulsifier for oil-in-water formulations.

steareth-21—an emulsifier most often employed in oil-in-water emulsions. Used in creams and lotions of all types, it serves to stabilize the emulsion and prevent separation of water and oils. It may also be used as a surfactant with very minor irritation to the skin and eyes.

stearic acid—an emulsifier and thickening agent found in many vegetable fats. Stearic acid is the main ingredient used in making bar soaps and lubricants. It occurs naturally in butter acids, tallow, cascarilla bark, and in other animal fats and oils. Stearic acid may cause allergic reactions in people with sensitive skin and is considered somewhat comedogenic. *See also* essential fatty acid entry in chapter 4.

stearic acid diethanolamide—*see* stearamide DEA.

stearoxy dimethicone—an emollient and skin-conditioning agent. *See also* dimethicone.

stearyl alcohol—used in cosmetic formulations for emulsions and antifoaming and lubricating action. Stearyl alcohol is also a viscosity agent and builder. It is a saturated alcohol of high purity.

stearyl heptanoate—a nongreasy emollient that produces a highly water-repellent film. Stearyl heptanoate is a natural preen gland wax.

sterols—a steroid alcohol that can be used as a lubricant in a variety of cosmetic preparations. Such alcohols contain the common steroid nucleus. Sterols are widely distributed in plants and animals, both in the free form and esterified to fatty acids. Cholesterol is a most important sterol and is often used in cosmetic creams. Ergosterol is an important plant sterol.

stinging nettle extract—traditionally used in mild acne conditions. *See also* nettle extract.

strawberry extract *(Fragaria vesca)*—considered astringent when the extract is obtained from the root. The fruit, in addition to malic and citric acids, sugar, mucilage, pectin, woody fiber, and water, also contains ascorbic acid that lends credence to early claims of bleaching properties. Extract from the fruit was recommended for use on sunburned areas to soothe the skin. Both the leaves and the fruit were in early pharmacopoeias; however there is no scientific evidence of benefit or harm.

sucrose (AKA table sugar)—an emollient, mild emulsifier, and humectant. It can be used in place of glycerin.

sucrose stearate—an emollient and emulsifying agent used primarily in makeup preparations. Sucrose stearate enables the formulation of clear gel microemulsion systems with a reduced physiological effect on the skin and eyes.

sulfated castor oil—a surfactant used as a cleansing agent.

sulfur—a mild antiseptic that is used in acne creams and lotions. Stimulates healing when used on skin rashes. May cause skin irritation. *See also* sulfur (colloidal).

sulfur (colloidal)—reduces oil-gland activity and dissolves the skin's surface layer of dry, dead cells. This ingredient is commonly used in acne soaps and lotions and is a major component in many acne preparations. It can cause allergic skin reactions in some sensitive people.

sulisobenzone (AKA benzophenone 4)—one of the 21 FDA-approved sunscreen chemicals with an approved usage level of 5–10%. It is considered a UVA absorber and is commonly used.

sumac extract *(Rhus glabra)* (AKA sumach)—astringent, anti-septic, and tonic properties are attributed to this botanical. Depending on the variety of sumac employed, extracts for skin problems are either made from the bark or the leaves. They may also be used for eczema and skin diseases. There are several varieties of this plant, some of which are poisonous. Those that are poisonous cause swelling, inflammation, and pain, ending in ulceration at the touch.

sumach—*see* sumac extract.

Sunarome OMC—a trade name for a sunscreen line.

sunflower oil *(Helianthus annuus)*—commonly used as a carrier oil. It has smoothing properties and is considered a noncomedogenic raw material. Sunflower oil has a high linoleic acid and essential fatty acid content. It also contains lecithin, carotenoids, and waxes.

sunflower seed oil—expressed from sunflower seeds. *See also* sunflower oil.

superoxide dimutase (AKA SOD)—an enzyme that can serve as an inhibitor of free radical production and a free radical scavenger. In cells it constitutes a natural defense system against activated oxygen species. SOD converts superoxide radical into hydrogen peroxide, which is then changed into molecular oxygen and water.

superoxide dimutase (polyoxyalkylene-modified)—used in cosmetic preparations to prevent drying and aging of the skin without causing irritation. *See also* superoxide dimutase.

sweet almond oil—an emollient with soothing properties. *See also* almond oil.

sweet clover extract—*see* clover extract.

sweet lime oil—*see* lime oil.

sweet marjoram oil *(Origanum majorana)*—the volatile oil distilled from the leaves of *Origanum majorana. See also* marjoram.

sweet orange extract—*see* orange extract.

synthetic spermaceti—*see* cetyl palmitate; spermaceti.

table salt—*see* sodium chloride.

table sugar—*see* sucrose.

talc—adds softness and sliding ability to a cosmetic formulation. Talc is also used as a bulking and opacifying agent, and it is used as an absorbent in makeup preparations. This is an inert powder, generally made from finely ground magnesium silicate, a mineral.

tallow—considered an occlusive skin-conditioning agent. Tallow is used primarily in the manufacture of soaps. It is the fat derived from the fatty tissue of sheep or cattle and is considered comedogenic.

tallow glycerides—a surfactant used as an emulsifying agent. Used more in makeup than skin care preparations. A mixture of triglycerides derived from tallow. *See also* tallow.

tangerine oil *(Citrus reticulata)*—has botanical properties similar to those of orange, though with greater antispasmodic and sedative properties. Its fragrance, reminiscent of bergamot, is sweeter than that of orange. *See also* orange oil.

tapioca flour *(Manihot utilissima* or *Jatropha manihot)*—used as a thickener. This is a starch derived from cassava.

tarragon *(Artemisia dracunculus)*—said to have tonic and stimulating properties. Its primary active is estragol, a phenol also known as methyl chavicol. Other constituents include cymene and phellandrene.

TEA (AKA triethanolamine)—an emulsifier and pH adjuster.

TEA dodecyl benzene sulfonate—a surfactant often mixed with other surfactants as a cleansing agent.

TEA isostearate—classified as a soap. This ingredient is a surfactant used as a cleansing and emulsifying agent.

TEA lactate—a surfactant.

TEA lauryl sulfate—a surfactant used as a cleansing agent with a moderate level of skin irritancy.

TEA oleamide PEG 2 sulfosuccinate—a surfactant with a very low level of skin irritancy.

TEA oleate—a mild emulsifier and surfactant.

TEA salicylate—a chemical UVB absorber. This is one of the 21 FDA-approved sunscreen chemicals with an approved usage level of 5–12%. TEA Salicylate is a water-soluble chemical with limited UV absorption capability. It is used in gels and hair products.

TEA stearate—a surfactant classified as an emulsifying and cleansing agent. TEA stearate is also a moisture absorber used in making emulsions. It may be irritating to the skin.

tea extract—studies are showing tea to have therapeutic effects, including antioxidation, bacteriostatic, and an antiallergenic action. Green tea extract in particular has been noted to be rich in potent antioxidants called catechins. Tea extract has been effectively used in eye treatment products to reduce puffiness.

tea tree oil *(Melaleuca alternifolia)* (AKA Australian tea tree oil)—considered a natural preservative with antiseptic, germicidal, and expectorant properties. Its antimicrobial activity toward a wide array of bacteria allows it to promote healing. It is becoming recognized as a topical remedy for yeast, fungus, and skin disorders and infections. Tea tree oil exhibits positive benefit against seborrhea, psoriasis (reduces scaling and redness), eczema (stops itching and reduces redness), and dermatitis. It has been used by Australian Aborigines to treat cuts, wounds, and skin infections and by European explorers as an herbal tea. This oil's ability to dissolve pus without causing visible or apparent damage to the skin's surface was noted by doctors when using it to clean the surface of infected wounds. It is also ideal for aromatherapy given its low toxicity. Though effectively used on almost any skin type, except sensitive or couperose skins, it is particularly beneficial to acne, problem, and/or congested skins. Tea tree oil is obtained from distilling the tree's leaves to produce a pale yellow to colorless oil that has a camphorlike scent similar to eucalyptus. Studies indicate it to be nontoxic with negligible to no irritancy.

tepescohuite —*see* mimosa tenuiflora.

4-tertbutyl 4'-methoxy-dibenzoylmethane — s*ee* butyl-methoxy dibenzoylmethane.

tetrahydroxypropyl ethylenediamine—used as a solvent and preservative. A component of the bacteria-killing substance in sugar cane. It is very alkaline. This ingredient may be irritating to the skin and mucous membranes and may cause skin sensitizations.

tetrasodium EDTA—used as a preservative and also as a sequestering and chelating agent in cosmetic solutions.

tetterwort extract *(Sanguinaria canadensis)* (AKA bloodroot)—herbal lore cites external application as helpful in treatment of eczema and other skin problems. The rootstock is the part used.

theophylline—a smooth muscle relaxant. Its current use in cosmetics has not been clearly established. Occurs in tea.

thiamine HCL (AKA vitamin B$_1$)—used as an emollient. *See also* vitamin B.

thuja extract—credited with healing and anti-irritant properties. It is potentially effective against pigmentation. The oil is obtained by distillation of small branches and twigs of yellow or white cedar. *See also* cedarwood oil.

thyme extract (*Thymus* sp.)—its botanical properties have been listed as antiseptic, tonic, anti bacterial, deodorizing, fungicidal, and circulation stimulating. Thyme extract may also have insect repellent properties. Its active principle is thymic acid, which has disinfectant properties similar to those of carbolic acid. Thyme extract may cause skin irritation.

thyme oil—considered a powerful antiseptic and tonic. Thyme oil serves as a natural preservative with antibacterial activity against a wide spectrum of bacterial classes. It has been widely used in botanical therapy since antiquity for its warming, stimulating and cleansing properties. The genus *Thymus* produces a variety of species, subspecies, and chemotypes, many with completely different chemical compositions. This includes citriodora thyme, lemon thyme, and red thyme. Lemon thyme is also described as healing and soothing for its use in skin care, while red thyme may cause skin irritation at high concentrations. The oil is obtained from the herb's branches and flowers.

thymus extract—according to some sources it improves cellular oxygenation and function. According to others it is a marketing and promotional tool with no proof of cellular benefit. It is an animal derived ingredient.

tilia (AKA linden)—botanical properties are described as antiseptic, soothing, and emollient. *See also* linden extract.

TiO$_2$—*see* titanium dioxide.

tissue respiratory factor (TRF) (AKA live yeast cell derivative)—described by manufacturers as a powerful anti-inflammatory and moisturizing agent that can promote wound healing. TRF is found to deliver its moisturizing, skin-soothing benefits more effectively than the traditional cosmetic raw materials. It also works with the skin to help improve the skin's appearance and overall health. It is obtained by stimulating living cells into producing protective substances. TRF can be described as a glyconucleopeptide and has been safely used for more than 40 years.

tissulan—a tissue extract with a high amino acid content. Claimed to improve the skin's surface and structure. *See also* amino acid.

titanium dioxide (AKA TiO$_2$)—a nonchemical SPF contributor. Titanium dioxide is one of the 21 FDA-approved sunscreen chemicals with an approved usage level of 2–25%. When applied, titanium dioxide remains on the skin's surface basically scattering UV light. It is often used in conjunction with other sunscreen chemicals to boost the product's SPF value, thus reducing the risk of irritation or allergies attributed to excessive usage of chemical sunscreens. Its incorporation into sunscreen formulations, makeup bases, and daytime moisturizers is dependent on the particular size of titanium dioxide employed. The smaller the particle size, the more unobtrusive its application. Large particles leave a whitish wash or look on the skin. Some companies list "micro" or "ultra" as a reference to the size of the titanium dioxide particle. According to some sources titanium dioxide could be the ideal UVA/UVB protection component given its chemical, cosmetic, and physical characteristics.

Titanium dioxide is also used to provide a white color to cosmetic preparations.

titanium dioxide (micro)—*see* titanium dioxide.

titanium dioxide (ultra)—*see* titanium dioxide.

tocopherol (AKA vitamin E)—an antioxidant obtained by vacuum distillation of edible vegetable oils. *See also* vitamin E.

tocopherol acetate—an antioxidant that helps prevent unsaturated oils and sebum from becoming rancid. It is considered a noncomedogenic raw material. *See also* vitamin E.

tocopherol ester—considered an effective free radical scavenger.

tocopherol nicotinate—used as an antioxidant and a skin-conditioning agent.

tocopheryl linoleate—used as an antioxidant and a skin-conditioning agent.

tocopheryl sorbate—most likely used as an antioxidant. This is a modified form of tocopherol. *See also* vitamin E; vitamin E acetate.

tomato oil—there is no evidence that tomato oil or its derivative compounds have any value when applied to the skin's surface. However, some sources cite it as being appropriate for combination skin.

tormentil extract *(Potentilla tormentilla)*—considered one of the safest and most powerful herbal astringents. It also has mildly antiseptic and anti-inflammatory properties. Used in Old England for sores, wounds, bruises, and infections. Important constituents of tormentil extract include tannin, phytosterols, flavonoids, chinovic acid, tormentoside, and pseudosaponine. The extract is obtained from the plant's root.

trace elements (AKA micronutrients; oligoelements)—different elements, usually inorganic, are considered essential to plant and animal nutrition in trace concentrations. The value of their topical application through cosmetic preparations is not clear, though some sources indicate a potential moisturization value.

trace element complex—*see* trace elements.

tragacanth gum—an effective emulsifying agent, also used as a stabilizing ingredient in lotion.

transglutaminase—an enzyme said to activate the skin's physiological functions.

tricaprylin—a skin-conditioning agent. *See also* caprylic/capric triglyceride.

triclosan—a preservative considered to have a low sensitizing potential in leave-on preparations.

tricontanyl PVP—a film-forming, waterproofing, and wear-proofing agent. It is oil soluble and easily formulated into sunscreens, skin care creams, lotions, and general cosmetic products. Tricontanyl PVP is a very versatile ingredient. When used in sunscreens, it facilitates the formulation of high SPFs without the need to significantly increase the use of sunscreen chemicals. The result is products with higher SPF, less or lower irritancy, and more cost effectiveness. Tricontanyl PVP is also used as a pigment dispersant in color cosmetics and is particularly useful when titanium dioxide is used to increase SPF values. Studies indicate little to no photoallergy or toxicity.

tridecyl stearate—a skin-conditioning agent and an emollient.

tridecyl trimelliatate—an occlusive skin-conditioning agent.

triethanolamine—*see* TEA.

triethanolamine oleate—*see* TEA oleate.

triethanolamine salicylate—*see* TEA salicylate.

triethanolamine stearate—*see* TEA stearate.

triethylene glycol—a solvent prepared from ethylene oxide and ethylene glycol.

triglycerides—consistency regulators for creams, lotions, and makeup. Facilitates skin blending and imparts good flow properties to products. These are the chief constituents of fats and oils. Fatty acids such as caprylic, capric, and lauric react with glycerin to produce triglyceride oils. These oils, such as those of almond, safflower, and cocoa butter, are utilized in cosmetics for enhanced lubricity and emolliency of a product. There are a variety of triglycerides, including caprylic/capric, lauric, myristic, palmitic, and stearic.

triisostearin—*see* glyceryl tri-isostearate.

triisostearyl citrate—an occlusive skin-conditioning agent. This is the triester of isostearyl alcohol and citric acid.

triisostearyl trilinoleate—a skin-conditioning and viscosity-increasing agent with occlusive properties.

trilinolein—a skin-conditioning and viscosity-increasing agent with occlusive properties.

trimethyl siloxy silicate—in combination with dimethicone it works as a waterproofing material for sunscreen preparations. It also reduces skin whitening and greasiness commonly associated with high SPF sunscreen formulations.

trisodium EDTA—a preservative. *See also* tetrasodium EDTA.

trisodium HEDTA (AKA trisodium hydroxy EDTA)—a preservative. *See also* tetrasodium EDTA.

trisodium hydroxy EDTA—*see* trisodium HEDTA.

trolamine —*see* triethanolamine.

tropocollagen—sometimes known as soluble collagen. It has excellent moisture-binding properties and forms a moisture-retentive film on the skin. Formulations using tropocollagen instead of regular collagen are reported to provide a smoother, silkier afterfeel on the skin. The fibroblast produces tropocollagen, which after aging is polymerized into collagen. Tropocollagen is obtained from animal connective tissues. *See also* collagen.

tropoelastin (AKA soluble elastin)—apparently it can compensate for the loss of (and aging of) the skin's own elastin. Reported to be more effective when applied on the skin than regular elastin. *See also* elastin.

tryptophan—one of the 21 amino acids comprising a protein. Tryptophan is a component of the skin's natural moisturizing factors. *See also* amino acid.

***l*-tyrosine**—experiments conducted with *l*-tyrosine in the form of water-soluble derivatives proved that it penetrates the epidermis to the basal layer where the melanocytes are located. Used in suntan accelerators and in skin bronzing cosmetics to accelerate the tanning process.

tyrosine—an amino acid. Cutaneous applications may produce an extra reserve of tyrosine in the skin, assisting or "activating" melanin synthesis. This in turn should increase and prolong the effect of the tanning process. Tyrosine's effect is improved if the product contains vitamin B (riboflavin) plus an additional compound referred to chemically as ATP (adenosine triphosphate). *See also* *l*-tyrosine.

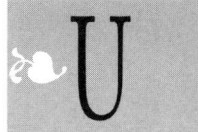

UVA screen (oil soluble)—a method of indicating that a given product contains sunscreen against UVA without revealing which or of what type. Refer to sunscreen entry in chapter 4.

UVB screen (oil soluble)—a method of indicating that a given product contains sunscreen against UVB without revealing which or of what type. Refer to sunscreen entry in chapter 4.

ultramarine blue—a color additive. Ultramarines can also be green, pink, red, or violet and are synthetic pigments composed of complex sodium aluminum sulfosilicated with the proportions of each element varying in each color. It was originally obtained naturally from ground lapis but is now produced synthetically. Used primarily in eye shadows, mascaras, and face powders. *See also* color entry in chapter 4.

ulve extract—*see* seaweed extract.

ulve seaweed—*see* seaweed extract.

undecylenoyl PEG 5 paraben—a preservative.

urea—found to increase absorption of other active ingredients, relieve itchiness, and help leave the skin feeling soft and supple. Urea is regarded as a "true" moisturizer rather than a humectant since it attracts and retains moisture in the corneum layer. It has a desquamating action as it dissolves intercellular cement in the corneum layer. Urea's incorporation into a product can also result in a lower use of other preservatives since urea can act as an antimicrobial given its ability to inhibit the growth of microorganisms. This ability is due to its property of water inclusion in its crystal structures. It can also regulate the hydrolipid mantle, considered a buffering action. Urea's properties include enhancing the penetration abilities of other active substances. Anti-inflammatory, antiseptic, and deodorizing actions allow it to protect the skin's surface against negative changes and help maintain healthy skin. Studies show that urea does not induce photoallergy, phototoxicity, or sensitization. The safest concentration of use in skin care preparations is between 2% and 8%. High concentrations of urea seem to be unstable when incorporated into skin care preparations and can also be irritating. Acidic urea solutions can produce burning or stinging sensations.

UV absorber 3—*see* 2-ethylhexyl 2-cyano-3, 3-diphenylacrylate.

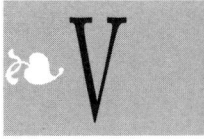

valerian oil *(Valeriana officinalis)*—considered a strong stimulant and antispasmodic oil with soothing effects. It is reported that when used frequently and in large quantities, valerian oil will produce headaches. The plant was held in such esteem as a remedy during medieval times that it was called All Heal. Its composition is complex, with constituents including valerianic, formic, and acetic acids; borneol (the alcohol); and pinene. The oil is present in the dried root in quantities of 0.5–2% depending on the plant variety and place of growth.

valeric acid—Obtained from valerian extract. *See also* valerian oil.

valine—an amino acid used as a skin-conditioning agent. It is more commonly used in hair care preparations than in skin care.

vanilla oil *(Vanilla planifolia)*—obtained from the cured, full-grown, unripe fruit of vanilla. It may cause a skin reaction in overly sensitive skin.

vanilla resinoid—a component of a natural preservative mixture that also includes linalool, ex-*bois de rose, bois de rose,* lemongrass, cedarwood oil, neroli bigarde petals oil, and other such exotic components.

Vaseline fluid—*see* petrolatum.

veegum—*see* magnesium aluminum silicate.

vegetable glyceride (hydrogenated)—an emollient and emulsifying agent obtained from vegetable oil. The oil source in this case is not identifiable.

vegetable oil—a carrier and an occlusive skin-conditioning agent. Such a listing may refer to a variety of oils alone or in combination, including peanut, corn, sesame, olive, and cottonseed. As the exact type of oil is not specified when listed in this fashion, it is difficult to determine the ingredient value or any skin reactions that may arise from the ingredient's use. Vegetable oil is an expressed oil of vegetable origin consisting primarily of triglycerides of fatty acids.

vegetable starch—a thickener.

verbena—*see* vervain oil.

veronica extract *(Veronica officinalis)*—credited with anti-inflammatory, healing, purifying, tonic, and soothing properties. Some say it promotes healthy tissue growth and a refinement of the pores. There are many species of veronica, with about 20 having been medicinally employed.

vervain oil *(Verbena officinalis)* (AKA verbena)—has been credited with astringent and antispasmodic properties. It is a perennial bearing many small, pale lilac flowers.

vetiver oil *(Vetiveria zizanioides)* (AKA khus-khus)—considered stimulant and tonic and is used in perfumery as well as in cosmetics. The oil, which has an aromatic to harsh woodsy odor, is produced from the roots of a fragrant grass.

violet extract *(Viola* sp.)—traditionally used for soothing and anti-itching skin treatments and as an antiseptic in skin creams and burn preparations. Violet extract also has cleansing properties. Its important constituents include saponins and salycic compounds. The extract has a slightly sweet, floral scent. While the violet family is comprised of over 200 species, it is the sweet-scented violet that appears to be most appropriate for botanical use. Violet extract may produce skin rash in those allergic to this particular plant.

vitamin A—can act as a keratinization regulator, helping to improve the skin's texture, firmness, and smoothness. Though not scientifically proven, it is believed that vitamin A esters, once in the skin, convert to retinoic acid and provide antiaging benefits. Vitamin A is believed to be essential for the generation and function of skin cells. Continued vitamin A deficiency shows a degeneration of dermal tissue, and the skin becomes thick and dry. Surface application of vitamin A helps prevent skin dryness and scaliness, keeping the skin healthy, clear, and infection resistent. Its skin regenerating properties appear enhanced when combined with vitamin E. Vitamins A and D are often used together in topical preparations. It has been claimed that this combination will stimulate epithelial growth and promote healthy healing of burned skin areas. Vitamin A is a major constituent of such oils as cod liver and shark and many fish and vegetable oils. *See also* retinol.

vitamin A palmitate—known as a skin "normalizer." It acts as an antikeratinizing agent, helping the skin stay soft and plump and improving its water-barrier properties. It is also an antioxidant. Because of its impact on the skin's water-barrier properties, it is useful against dryness, heat, and pollution. It is also suggested for use in sunscreens. Clinical studies with vitamin A palmitate indicate a significant change in skin composition, with increase in collagen, DNA, skin thickness, and elasticity. Vitamin A palmitate's stability is superior to retinol.

vitamin B—the literature tends to indicate that B vitamins cannot pass through the layers of the skin and hence are of no value in the skin surface. Current experiments are demonstrating, however, that vitamin B_2 acts as a chemical reaction accelerator, enhancing the performance of tyrosine derivatives in suntan-accelerating preparations. *See also* panthenol for B_5; pyridoxine tripalmitate for B_6; riboflavin for B_2; thiamine HCL for vitamin B_1.

vitamin C—considered the most important water-soluble antioxidant. Although vitamin C has antioxidant properties, it has not been clearly determined that its application on the skin surface as part of a cream will have an internal effect on free radical formation. The effectiveness of topical applications has been questioned due to vitamin C's instability (it reacts with water and degrades). Some forms are said to have better stability in water systems. Synthetic analogues such as magnesium ascorbyl phosphate are among those considered more effective as they tend to be more stable. Researchers claim that treatments with topically applied vitamin C inhibit UVA and UVB radiation-induced damage. The current research also indicates that high concentrations of topically applied vitamin C are photoprotective, and apparently the vitamin preparation used in these studies resists soap-and-water washing or rubbing for three days. This would lead one to conclude that in combination with conventional sunscreen chemicals, vitamin C may allow for longer-lasting, broader sun protection. Vitamin C also acts as a collagen biosynthesis regulator. It is known to control intercellular colloidal substances such as collagen, and, when formulated into the proper vehicles, it can have a skin-lightening effect. It is said to be able to help the body fortify against infectious conditions by strengthening the immune system. There is some evidence (though debated) that vitamin C can pass through the layers of the skin and promote healing of tissue damaged by burns or injury. It is found, therefore, in burn ointments and creams used for abrasions. Current studies indicate possible anti-inflammatory properties as well. *See also* ascorbic acid.

vitamin D—acts as a keratinization regulator, helping to improve skin feel and firmness with repeated use. This vitamin is absorbed through the skin's outer layers. Studies are indicating that vitamin D is an important factor in epidermal cell turnover. It is generally found in combination with vitamin A as such a mixture appears to help epithelial growth and good pigmentation. Like vitamin A, vitamin D is a major constituent of many fish and vegetable oils.

vitamin E (AKA D-alpha-tocopherol; DL-alpha-tocopherol; tocopherol)—considered the most important oil-soluble antioxidant and free radical scavenger. Studies indicate that vitamin E performs these functions when applied topically. It is also a photoprotectant, and it helps protect the cellular membrane from free radical damage. In addition, vitamin E serves a preservative function due to its ability to protect against oxidation. This benefits not only the skin, but also the product in terms of longevity. As a moisturizer vitamin E is well absorbed through the skin, demonstrating a strong affinity with small blood vessels. It is also considered to improve the skin's water-binding ability. In addition, vitamin E emulsions have been found to reduce transepidermal water loss, thereby improving the appearance of rough, dry, and damaged skin. This vitamin is also believed to help maintain the connective tissue. There is also evidence that vitamin E is effective in preventing irritation due to sun exposure. Many studies show that vitamin E topically applied prior to UV irradiation is protective against epidermal cell damage caused by inflammation. This indicates possible anti-inflammatory properties. Lipid peroxidation in tissues may be one cause of skin aging. Vitamin E, however, appears to counteract decreased functioning of the sebaceous glands and reduce excessive skin pigmentation, which is found to increase almost linearly with age. Vitamin E is very unstable. It is available also as a tocopherol-polypeptide complex that delivers the vitamin in a water-dispersable form. In this way, when incorporated into cosmetic formulations, it does not need other compounds to assist in its solubilization. Useful in antiaging creams and lotions and in UV protective products, tocopherol is a naturally occurring vitamin E found in a variety of cereal germ oils, including wheat germ oil. It can also be produced synthetically. *See also* acetate.

vitamin E acetate (AKA tocopherol acetate)—an antioxidant with skin-moisturizing properties. Given its free radical scavenging properties, it is useful in UV protective products. Vitamin E acetate is commonly used to replace vitamin E because it is more stable and is converted to vitamin E by the body. *See also* vitamin E.

vitamin E linoleate—a synthetic version of vitamin E. *See also* tocopheryl linoleate; vitamin E.

vitamin F—used in the treatment and care of dry skin. *See also* arachidonic acid; linoleic acid; linolenic acid.

vitamin H—*see* biotin.

vitamin P—considered a vascular protector. Reported to increase resistance to collagen destruction.

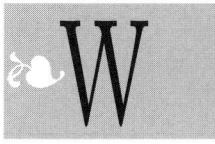

walnut extract (*Juglans* sp.)—traditionally used topically for soothing and anti-itching as well as against sunburns and other superficial burns. It can be used in cases of acne and skin diseases because of it fungistatic and astringent properties. Though extracts are obtained from the leaves and bark, the oil is extracted from the ripe nut.

walnut meal—a mild abrasive.

walnut shell meal—an abrasive.

walnut shell powder—used as an abrasive and bulking agent in cleansers, scrubs, soaps, and masks. It is the powder ground from the shell of English walnuts.

water—listed also as catalyzed, deionized, demineralized, distilled, pure spring, and purified water. Water is an important skin component and is essential for its proper functioning. It is the most common ingredient used in cosmetic formulations and therefore is generally listed first on product labels. Water is usually processed to eliminate hardness and minerals and to avoid product contamination.

watercress extract *(Nasturtium officinale)*—used in folklore for cleansing external ulcers and in night creams for freckles, spots, and acne. It is believed to help reduce sebum production. Watercress extract is utilized as a moisture regulator and skin activator for sunburn (and bath) preparations. Important constituents of watercress include minerals, flavonoids, and vitamins. This is a hardy perennial found in abundance near springs and open running watercourses.

wax (self-emulsifying)—can be obtained from insects, animals, and plants like roses, and each has its own set of characteristics. Beeswax, for example, is glossy and hard but changes to a plastic texture when warm. Wax esters, such as lanolin or spermaceti, are less greasy, harder, and more brittle than fats. Waxes are generally nontoxic to the skin but, depending on their source, may cause allergic reactions in some sensitive people.

wheat bran extract—considered a moisturizer due to its carbohydrate/sugar components. This is the extract from the broken coat material of wheat grains.

wheat germ extract—used in cosmetics because of its large vitamin E content. This extract is obtained from the wheat kernel embryo separated in milling. *See also* vitamin E.

wheat germ glycerides—softens the skin and has good penetration ability. Commonly used in moisturizers in concentrations of 0.1–5%. Wheat germ glycerides contain polyunsaturated fats, key for healthy skin. This is a mixture of mono-, di-, and triglycerides produced by the transesterification of wheat germ oil. Although some sources indicate it as having an irritancy potential, safety tests show it to be nonsensitizing and nonirritating to the skin. It is considered by some to be somewhat comedogenic.

wheat germ oil—an emollient with antioxidant and free radical scavenging properties due to its vitamin E content. Another important constituent of wheat germ oil is lecithin. The oil is obtained by the expression or extraction of wheat germ. *See also* tocopherol; vitamin E.

wheat germ oil (unsaponifiable)—acts as a hormonelike cellular messenger targeting epidermal keratinocytes, particularly the dermal fibroblast. It is said in studies that this results in a stimulation of the fibroblast to produce collagen, elastin, proteoglycans, and structural glycoproteins.

wheat protein—has elastic and-binding properties, helps reduce the irritating effect of surfactants, and, apparently, demonstrates excellent emulsifying action. As it forms a film on the skin's surface it also moisturizes and conditions the skin, increasing skin firmness by helping minimize transepidermal water loss. Some forms of wheat protein are said to be able to penetrate down into the wrinkles and superficial hollows of the skin, forming a film that contracts upon drying, causing the flattening out of the skin and a reduction in surface roughness.

wheat protein (soluble)—*see* wheat protein.

wheat starch—used as a demulcent and emollient and in face powders. Wheat starch swells when water is added. It is obtained from wheat.

white clover—*see* melilot.

white dead-nettle—*see* white nettle.

white lily bulb extract *(Lilium candidum)* (AKA Madonna lily)—has antiseptic and soothing properties. The roots contain tannin, gallic acid, mucilage, starch, gum, resin, sugar, ammonia, tartaric acid, and fecula. This is a perennial aquatic herb that grows to the surface of the water from a thick horizontal rootstock.

white nettle *(Lamium album)* (AKA white dead-nettle)—considered astringent. It is obtained from the plant's flowers. *See also* nettle.

313

white willow extract *(Salix alba)*—deodorant with tonic and astringent properties. It is used effectively in products for acne and eczema. The extract is obtained from the bark of this large tree, which contains tannin as a chief constituent and a small quantity of salicin. *See also* willow extract.

wild alum—astringent and deodorant. It is cited as good for oily skin.

wild marjoram—*see* wild Spanish marjoram.

wild pansy extract—*see* pansy extract.

wild Spanish marjoram (AKA wild marjoram)—described as having antiseptic and anti-inflammatory botanical properties. *See also* marjoram.

wild thyme extract *(Thymus serpyllum)*—an emollient, tonic, and antiseptic extract traditionally used to clean wounds after washing. Believed not to be as effective as the common thyme variety. It contains 30–70% phenols—thymol, carvacrol, etc. When distilled, some 225 pounds of dried material yield 150 grams of essence. Wild thyme is a perennial herb.

willow extract *(Salix sp.)*—described as antiseptic and skin clearing. The roots and leaves have demulcent, tonic, and astringent properties. Apparently it is very mild, hence its incorporation in lotions and creams for infants.

winterbloom infusion—*see* witch hazel.

witch hazel distillate—an aqueous solution obtained by distillation of *Hamamelis virginiana* twigs. *See also* witch hazel extract.

witch hazel extract *(Hamamelis virginiana)* (AKA hamamelis; winterbloom)—traditionally used in topical treatment of burns, sunburns, skin irritation, insect bites, and bruises. It is credited with anti-inflammatory and wound-healing properties. It is often used for its anti-itching, softening, and emollient properties. In addition, witch hazel is being found effective against free radicals and is being used in solar products. It apparently counters the effects of UVA by its anti-free radical activity while acting as a UVA and UVB absorber. Ideal applications for witch hazel are in sun preparations, aftersun preparations, and creams that strive to regenerate overstrained skin. It can be formulated effectively into gels as an antiseptic preparation for treating impure, greasy skin. Some sources cite a recommended dosage of 2–5% for use in formulations. Obtained from the leaves and bark of the plant.

wood alcohol—*see* alcohol.

wood sage—*see* germander extract.

wool wax alcohols—*see* lanolin alcohol.

woundwort extract *(Stachys sylvatica* and *Stachys palustris)*—in herbal medicine it is considered antiseptic, astringent, and tonic. The extract, obtained from the leaves, has been credited with stopping bleeding and healing wounds.

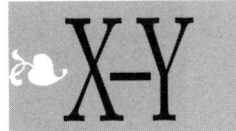

xanthan gum (AKA corn starch gum)—serves as a texturizer, carrier agent, and gelling agent in cosmetic preparations. It also stabilizes and thickens formulations. This is the gum produced through a fermentation of carbohydrate and *Anthomonas camestris*.

yarrow extract *(Achillea millefolium)* (AKA *Achillea* extract; milfoil)—general effects attributed to yarrow include antiphilogistic and spasmolytic. It is famous in folkloric medicine for stopping the bleeding of wounds and nosebleeds. Studies indicate an antibiotic effect and an ability to reduce the blood's clotting time. Yarrow extract is also described as having astringent, antiseptic, anti-inflammatory, healing, and calming properties. Considered good in the care of oily and acne skins. Yarrow's important constituents include flavonoids, amino acids, sugars, and phytosterols. It grows everywhere, in grass, meadows, pastures, and by the roadside. Since it creeps by its roots and multiplies by its seeds, yarrow becomes a troublesome weed in gardens. The whole plant is used for making the extract.

yeast—has a rubefactant effect on the skin making it good for pale, yellow skins. It is used in face masks designed to give the skin a ruddy color. Yeast is a fungus whose usual and dominant growth form is unicelluar. It can be irritating to dry or sensitive skins. *See also* malt.

yeast extract—manufacturers claim it is able to revitalize the skin with moisture, fighting dryness and giving the skin a radiant appearance. In addition, it is claimed that yeast extract has the ability to minimize the dryness and pain associated with sunburned and wind-chapped skin; restore the comfort of soft, elastic, and healthy skin; reduce facial lines; and improve dry skin. Its constituents include enzymes, vitamins, sugars, and mineral substances. Though originally made exclusively from animal-derived materials such as blood serums, placenta extracts, and spleen extracts, some yeast cells derived from plant materials are now available to cosmetic formulators.

ylang-ylang extract—*see* ylang-ylang oil.

ylang-ylang oil *(Unona odorantissimum* and *Canaga odorata)*—used in folklore as a scenting agent and for insect bites. Ylang-ylang is found to be relaxing and an excellent antistress agent. In addition, it is credited with antiseptic, softening, smoothing, rejuvenating, calming, soothing, and antispasmodic properties. It is credited good for inflamed and/or irritated skin and for controlling acne. Ylang-ylang oil is said to help balance the skin and work to reduce oiliness. Along with its therapeutic effects, ylang-ylang is also believed effective for its tension relieving properties since a variety of skin disorders (e.g., acne and eczema) can be aggravated by stress. Some sources cite that it takes roughly 100 pounds of blossoms to produce about 2 pounds of essential oil. This oil is produced via steam distillation into a fragrant yellowish oil of varying grades.

ylang-ylang water—*see* ylang-ylang oil.

zinc—described as an oligoelement, trace element, or micronutrient. Zinc is believed to accelerate wound healing and offer protection against UV radiation. It appears to favor the sulfur uptake in sulfurated amino acids and facilitates the incorporation into the skin of the cystine amino acid. It also has a synergistic effect with vitamins A and E. A structural component or, at the very least, part of more than 70 metal enzymes, zinc promotes collagen synthesis in the dermis and keratinization of the corneum layer. Zinc is useful for acne treatments since it lowers sebaceous secretion and is also used in the treatment of psoriasis.

zinc aspartate—a skin-conditioning agent. Zinc aspartate is the zinc salt of aspartic acid.

zinc oxide—has been used to protect, soothe, and heal the skin. Zinc oxide provides an excellent barrier to the sun and other irritants. It is somewhat astringent, antiseptic, and antibactericidal. When used in sunscreen preparations, it can contribute to and/or increase SPF. It has UVA and UVB absorption characteristics. At the appropriate partical size zinc oxide is transparent in the visible light spectrum but opaque in the UV ranges, thereby avoiding a whitening effect when incorporated into sunscreen preparations. Zinc oxide is not yet included on the FDA's list of approved sunscreen chemicals, but it is expected to be included in Category I. This compound acts more like a UVA absorber and thus can boost SPF while providing UVA protection. Additionally, the use of zinc oxide may inhibit some technical formulation problems in emulsion stability. It is also used when a white color is desired for a product. Zinc oxide is obtained from zinc ore, a commonly found mineral, and is relatively nonallergenic.

zinc pyrithione—a preservative against bacteria, fungi, and yeast. It is unstable in light and in the presence of oxidyzing agents. Zinc pyrithione is useful in gels, creams, heavy lotions, and talcum powder.

zinc stearate—used in cosmetic formulations to increase adhesive properties. It is also used as a coloring agent. This is a mixture of the zinc salts of stearic and palmitic acids.

zinc sulfate—a cosmetic astringent and biocide produced through the reaction of sulfuric acid with zinc. It is irritating to the skin and mucous membranes and may cause an allergic reaction.

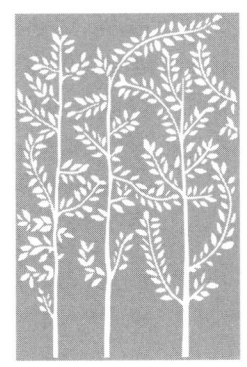

Appendix
BOTANICAL
LATIN NAMES

Acacia senegal—acacia
Achillea millefolium—milfoil, yarrow
Aesculus hippocastanum—horse chestnut
Agrimonia eupatoria—agrimony
Alchemilla vulgaris—alchemilla, lady's mantle
Aleurites moluccana—kukui nut oil
Allium sativum—garlic
Aloe vera—aloe vera
Alternifolia—see *Melaleuca alternifolia.*
Althaea officinalis—althea
Anemone sp.—anemone
Angelica sp.—angelica
Anthemis nobilis—Roman chamomile
Arboresenes artemesia—southernwood
Arctium lappa—burdock

Arctostaphylus uva-urusi—bearberry
Armoracia lapathifolia—horseradish
Arnica montana—arnica
Artemisia dracunculus—tarragon
Avena sativa—oat
Bellis perennis—daisy
Berberis vulgaris—barberry
Beta vulgaris—beet
Betula sp.—birch
Bixa orellana—annatto
Borago officinalis—borage
Boswellia thurifera—frankincense
Calamintha officinalis—calamint
Calendula officinalis—calendula
Canaga odorata—ylang-ylang
Carduus marianus—milk thistle
Carica papaya—papaya
Caroba balsam—carob
Carthamus tinctorius—safflower
Carum carvi—caraway
Caryophyllus aromaticus—clove
Castanea sativa—chestnut
Centaurea cyanus—cornflower
Centella asiatica—gotu kola
Certraria islandica—Iceland moss
Chondrus crispus—carrageen, Irish moss
Chrysanthemum parthenium—feverfew
Cinchona ledgeriana—cinchona
Cinnamomum camphora—camphor
Cinnamomum zeylanicum—cinnamon
Citrus acida—lime
Citrus aurantifolia—lime
Citrus aurantium—bitter orange, Italian orange

Citrus bergamia—bergamot
Citrus limonum—lemon extract
Citrus paradisi—grapefruit
Citrus reticulata—tangarine
Citrus sinensis—sweet orange
Cochlearia officinalis—scurvy grass
Cola acuminata—kola tree
Commiphora meccanensis—balm of Gilead
Commiphora opobalsamum—balm of Gilead
Commiphora myrrha—myrrh
Coriandrum sativum—coriander
Crataegus oxyacantha—hawthorn
Cucumis sativus—cucumber
Cupressus sp.—cypress
Cymbopogon citratus—lemongrass
Cymbopogon martini—palmarosa
Cynara scolymus—artichoke
Daucus carota—carrot
Echinacea angustifolia—echinacea
Elettaria cardamomum—cardamom
Equisetum arvense—horsetail
Eucalyptus globulus—eucalyptus
Euphrasia officinalis—eyebright
Evernia prunastri—oakmoss
Fagus sylvatica—beech
Filipendula ulmaria—meadowsweet
Foeniculum vulgare—fennel
Fragaria vesca—strawberry
Fucus vesiculosus—fucus seaweed
Fumaria officinalis—fumitory
Galium aparine—cleavers
Gentiana sp.—gentian
Geranium maculatum—crane's bill

Geum urbanum—avens
Ginkgo biloba—ginkgo
Glycyrrhiza glabra—licorice
Gnaphalium polycephalum—everlasting
Guaiacum officinale—guaiac
Hamamelis virginiana—witch hazel
Harpagophytum procumbens—devil's claw
Hedera helix—ivy
Helianthus annuus—sunflower
Hibiscus sp.—hibiscus
Hordeum vulgare—barley
Humulus lupulus—hops
Hydrastis canadensis—goldenseal
Hydrocotyl asiatica—gotu kola
Hypericum perforatum—St. John's wort
Hyssopus officinalis—hyssop
Inula helenium—elecampane
Iris sp.—iris
Jacaranda procera—carob
Jasminum officinale—jasmine
Jatropha manihot—tapioca
Juglans sp.—walnut
Juniperus communis—juniper
Lactuca virosa—lettuce
Laminaria digitata—seaweed
Lamium album—white nettle, blind nettle
Lamnanthes alba—meadowfoam
Laurus nobilis—laurel
Lavandula officinalis—lavender
Lawsonia inermis—henna
Levisticum officinale—lovage
Lilium candidum—white lily
Lonicera fragrantissima—honeysuckle

Lycopodium clavatum—club moss
Malva sylvestris—mallow
Macademia integrifolia—macadamia nut tree
Manihot utilissima—tapioca
Matricaria chamomilla—German chamomile
Medicago sativa—alfalfa
Melaleuca alternifolia—tea tree
Melaleuca leucadendron—cajeput
Melilotus officinalis—melilot
Melissa officinalis—balm mint
Mentha sp.—mint
Mentha piperita—peppermint
Mentha viridis—spearmint
Monarda didyma—bergamot
Myrica cerifera—bayberry
Myristica fragrans—nutmeg
Myrospermum toluiferum—balsam of tolu
Myroxylon pereirae—balsam of Peru
Nasturtium officinale—watercress
Ocimum basilicum—basil
Oenothera biennis—evening primrose
Olea europaea—olive
Ononis arvensis—restharrow
Ononis spinosa—restharrow
Orchis sp.—orchid
Origanum majorana—sweet marjoram
Origanum vulgare—marjoram
Oryza sativa—rice
Paeonia officinalis—peony
Panax sp.—ginseng
Papaver sp.—poppy
Papaver rhoeas—red poppy
Passiflora incarnata—passion flower

Pelargonium sp.—geranium
Petroselinum sativum—parsley
Phaseolus vulgaris—bean
Phoradendron flavescens—American mistletoe
Picea excelsa—spruce
Picraena excelsa—quassia
Pimpinella anisum—anise
Pinus sp.—pine
Plantago sp.—plantain
Pogostemon patchouli—patchouli
Potentilla anserina—cinquefoil
Potentilla tormentilla—tormentil
Primula officinalis—primula
Prunus persica—peach
Pyrola elliptica—shinleaf
Pyrus cydonia—quince
Pyrus malus—apple
Quercus sp.—oak
Rhamnus purshiana—casacara sagrada
Rhus glabra—sumac
Ribes nigrum—black currant
Ricinus communis—castor oil plant
Rosa sp.—rose
Rosmarinus officinalis—rosemary
Rubus idaeus—raspberry
Rubus villosus—blackberry
Rumex acetosa—sorrel
Ruscus aculeatus—butchersbroom
Salix sp.—willow
Salvia officinalis—sage
Salvia sclarea—clary sage
Sambucus sp.—elder
Sanguinaria canadensis—bloodroot, tetterwort

Santalum album—sandalwood
Saponaria officinalis—soapwort
Sassafras albidum—sassafras
Satureia hortensis—savory
Scrophularia nodosa—figwort
Simmondsis chinensis—jojoba
Smilax officinalis—sarsasparilla
Solidago sp.—goldenrod
Spireae ulmaria—meadowsweet
Stachys officinalis—betony
Stachys palustris—woundwort, marsh
Stachys sylvatica—woundwort, hedge
Symphytum officinale—comfrey
Syzygium aromaticum—clove
Taraxacum officinale—dandelion
Taraktogenos kurzii—chaulmoogra
Teucrium scorodonia—germander
Thuja occidentalis—cedar
Thymus sp.—thyme
Thymus serpyllum—wild thyme
Tilia sp.—linden
Trifolium sp.—clover
Trigonella foenumgraecum—fenugreek
Tropaeolum majus—nasturtium
Turnera aphrodisiaca—damiana
Tussilago farfara—coltsfoot
Ulmus sp.—elm
Ulmus fulva—slippery elm
Unona odorantissimum—ylang-ylang
Urtica dioica—nettle
Valeriana officinalis—valerian
Vanilla planifolia—vanilla
Verbena officinalis—vervain

Appendix

Veronica officinalis—veronica
Vetiveria zizanioides—vetiver, khus-khus
Viola sp.—violet
Viola tricolor—pansy
Viscum album—European mistletoe